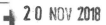

A GUIDE TO UNDERSTANDING AND DEALING WITH
DEMENTIA

What You Need to Know

Dr Keith Souter

Foreword by Professor Graham Stokes
Global Director of Dementia Care, Bupa

Vie Books is an imprint of Summersdale Publishers Ltd

Summersdale Publishers Ltd
46 West Street
Chichester
West Sussex
PO19 1RP
UK

www.summersdale.com

Printed and bound by CPI Group (UK) Ltd, Croydon, CR0 4YY

ISBN: 978-1-84953-770-4

Substantial discounts on bulk quantities of Summersdale books are available to corporations, professional associations and other organisations. For details contact Nicky Douglas by telephone: +44 (0) 1243 756902, fax: +44 (0) 1243 786300 or email: nicky@summersdale.com.

Disclaimer
Every effort has been made to ensure that the information in this book is accurate and current at the time of publication. The author and the publisher cannot accept responsibility for any misuse or misunderstanding of any information contained herein, or any loss, damage or injury, be it health, financial or otherwise, suffered by any individual or group acting upon or relying on information contained herein. None of the opinions or suggestions in this book are intended to replace medical opinion. If you have concerns about your health, please seek professional advice.

In memory of my grandfather, who taught me so much

And for my nephew, Simon, for his work with Alzheimer's Society

Acknowledgements

I would like to thank Isabel Atherton, my wonderful agent at Creative Authors, for helping to bring another book in this series to fruition. Thanks also to Claire Plimmer at Summersdale who commissioned this and the previous titles, and to Stephen Brownlee who has guided it through the various stages towards publication. Thanks to my editor, Jennifer Barclay. It was good to work with her again and I am grateful for the many helpful suggestions she made. Thanks also to Julian Beecroft, my copy editor, who helped to smooth out the manuscript, and Vicki McKay, my proofreader. It has been a great pleasure to work with them all.

Finally, a huge thank you to Professor Graham Stokes for taking the time from his busy schedule to write the foreword to this book. I particularly valued his opinion as a clinician and academic working in the field of dementia.

Keith Souter

Contents

Depression
Delirium
Hypothyroidism
B12 deficiency
Parkinson's disease
Deafness
Brain tumour
Charles Bonnet syndrome
Mild cognitive impaiment, MCI

Foreword

By Professor Graham Stokes
Global Director of Dementia Care, Bupa
Honorary Visiting Professor of Person-Centred Dementia Care, University of Bradford
Co-Chair, Dementia Action Alliance

In the United Kingdom the number of people with dementia is set to double over the next 35 years to reach nearly 1.75 million. Most will also be experiencing the ravages of advanced old age. There is no doubt this will exercise an unprecedented burden of responsibility on the NHS and caring services, yet this staggering increase in the numbers living with dementia, the most common cause of which is Alzheimer's disease, is no longer solely a concern for health officials, doctors and social services. Rather, as dementia touches every family in the land, there is a need for society to become more dementia aware, to become more dementia friendly, and embrace a personal and civic responsibility to be informed about not simply the nature of dementia, but also how to understand what it means to live with a condition of the brain that progressively destroys the ability to remember, speak and reason, and what it takes to care well for someone living with a condition that eventually destroys self-awareness – an understanding that embraces the knowledge that for both those who care and those who need to be cared for there is rarely any true respite.

If it is possible for a book to explain the nature of dementia and brain function, address the experiences that comprise living and coping with dementia, and how to navigate the labyrinthine world of health and social care, this one does. Through fifteen informative, engaging and accessible chapters Keith Souter provides knowledge and insights that embrace not only the pathology of dementia but brings the need to live well with dementia to the fore. Each chapter contributes to the weaving of a tapestry that successfully integrates biology, person and care to give an overview of a journey with dementia from what can be done to reduce risk, to getting a diagnosis, to eventually sound advice regarding the choice of a care home. Complex information is rendered meaningful and summarised as 'key points' providing the reader with an excellent overview of the diseases that cause dementia as well as what is not dementia but may appear so, and of great importance 'tips' on not only how to survive with dementia but how to be a person who confronts and rises above the emotional and practical challenges that confront all those affected. Throughout, this guide resonates with the need to be person-centred in all that is planned and provided.

I am in no doubt that the subject of this book is of increasing and pressing importance. All involved in the support and care of people with dementia, all who know someone who appears muddled and absent-minded whether that is a partner, relative, friend or neighbour, as well as those who are or fear they may be living with the beginnings of dementia will benefit from investing their time in reading this guide.

We are motivated to understand how we can help people with dementia and their carers have fulfilling lifestyles that truly reveal life is worth living. We should be grateful for this book.

Introduction

One of the greatest fears that most people have is that they may lose their mental function and end their days slipping into dementia. Many of us will have had a relative with dementia and seen a gradual deterioration in their mental and physical health. The idea of losing control of one's thoughts, memory and ability to communicate causes understandable anxiety.

Unfortunately, there is still a stigma about dementia. Inevitably, this makes people reluctant to talk about it, leading to a lot of ignorance on the subject. A result of this is that people who have dementia can feel isolated. Even worse, people who have memory problems or may be in the early stages of dementia can feel ashamed to have developed something that is stigmatised. This is something that we as a society have to work to overcome. The fact is, there is no shame at all in having dementia.

There is every need to keep people with dementia active and integrated into society. In this regard, being friends with people who have dementia, and having a supportive and caring attitude, can help them to deal with their condition.

Dementia is not a single condition, but an umbrella term used for a group of brain disorders that cause a deterioration of intellectual faculties such as memory, concentration and judgement. It is often accompanied by emotional disturbance and personality changes. The commonest form is Alzheimer's disease, which accounts for about 60–70 per cent of cases, followed by vascular dementia, which makes up about 20 per cent. We shall consider these and the other types later in the book.

Dementia has been observed in all societies and cultures throughout history. The name comes from the Latin *demens*, which means 'out of one's mind or senses', a bleak phrase that gives some idea why, in the past, people suffering from dementia were given so little help. They were left in the care of the family and, when the family could no longer deal with them, they might end up being admitted to a residential home or a psychiatric hospital. Treatment was often minimal, amounting to sedation with tranquillisers to keep them 'manageable'.

Fortunately, today there is growing recognition that a person with dementia can continue to live well and enjoy life. Well-known people, such as the novelist Sir Terry Pratchett among many others, have done much to show that they can still be useful and contribute to society even after a diagnosis has been made.

The diagnosis can be frightening for the individual, with the potential to have devastating consequences for the most important relationships in someone's life. Thus it is important to maintain the dignity of a person with dementia, to prevent them from simply being someone who receives care. Their uniqueness as an individual, their personal worth and their personal needs must always be of paramount importance. For this reason, a person-centred approach is what is needed.

The purpose of this book is to help the individual who may be experiencing memory problems, or who is concerned that they or a friend or relative might be developing dementia, by explaining the way the brain works and the various types of dementia, the tests that may lead to a diagnosis and the help that may be available. It also aims to dispel some of the myths that surround the condition. In addition, it will cover the treatments available and the strategies that can deal with the illness as it develops.

Part One

UNDERSTANDING DEMENTIA

Living well with dementia

In 2009 the UK government set out a National Dementia Strategy, called Living Well with Dementia.[1] This recognised that although dementia is a progressive condition that gets worse over time, people who have the condition can still have a good quality of life for several years.

The strategy is aimed at people with dementia as well as carers, health professionals and anyone who is affected by dementia. That may mean friends or relatives of someone with dementia.

There are three key steps in this strategy:

- Ensure better knowledge and understanding about dementia

- Ensure early diagnosis, support and treatment of people with dementia, and support for their family and carers

- Develop services to meet changing needs.

All of this is important. As dementia is becoming increasingly common, we must be prepared as a society to improve the care people receive and to ensure that people are enabled to live well with the condition. It is important to offer early diagnosis so that whatever supports are needed can be given.

Chapter 1

So what is dementia?

The World Health Organization uses the definition given by the International Classification of Diseases.[2]

Dementia is a syndrome due to disease of the brain – usually of a chronic or progressive nature – in which there is disturbance of multiple higher cortical functions, including memory, thinking, orientation, comprehension, calculation, learning capacity, language, and judgement. Consciousness is not clouded. The impairments of cognitive function are commonly accompanied, and occasionally preceded, by deterioration in emotional control, social behaviour, or motivation. This syndrome occurs in a large number of conditions primarily or secondarily affecting the brain.

The point about there being no impairment of consciousness is very important, since it can help to differentiate between dementia itself and potentially reversible conditions that may mimic the condition. This will be explained later.

There are over 200 types of dementia, but the most common according to figures from Alzheimer's Society are:

- Alzheimer's disease: the commonest – accounts for 62 per cent of cases of dementia

- Vascular dementia: the second commonest – 17 per cent

- Mixed pattern – 10 per cent

- Dementia with Lewy bodies – 4 per cent. It has characteristics of both Alzheimer's disease and Parkinson's disease and also Parkinson's disease dementia PDD

- Fronto-temporal dementia – 2 per cent

- Parkinson's disease dementia PDD – 2 per cent

- Others including Creutzfeldt-Jakob disease, Korsakoff's psychosis, and Huntington's disease.

Causes of dementia in the UK

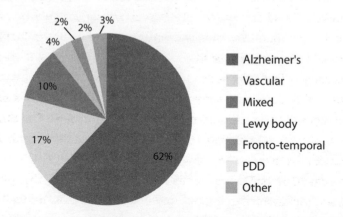

KEY POINT

Dementia is NOT a normal part of ageing.

A brief history of dementia

Dementia is not a new condition but has been recognised for centuries. It is instructive to consider how it has been regarded down the years and to see how we have gradually come to understand more about it. Thus we now realise that dementia is merely an umbrella label for a wide spectrum of brain disorders.

Ancient Egypt

The ancient Egyptians left us a great deal of information about their civilisation in tomb paintings and in the many papyri that have been discovered by archaeologists. In 1862, Edwin Smith, a young amateur Egyptologist and adventurer, purchased two papyri in Luxor, said to have been found between the legs of a mummy in the Theban necropolis. Both papyri dated to about 1550 BC, but were thought to be copies of far older texts. One is the oldest-known surgical text in the world, describing surgical instruments and techniques and discussing 48 cases of injuries, including head injuries. The other is a medical text outlining knowledge about medicine and the treatments used for a whole range of conditions.[3]

The Egyptians had hieroglyphics for the brain, the skull, the spinal fluid and the meninges, and the coverings of the brain, as well as for the other major organs. They knew that the brain was needed to control the movements of the body, and they recognised that injury to one side of the brain could result in paralysis of the opposite side of the body.

A beautiful and historically accurate description of ancient Egyptian surgery is given in the 1945 historical novel *The Egyptian* by the Finnish writer, Mika Waltari. The main character Sinuhe, who would become the royal physician to Pharaoh Akhenaten, is apprenticed to the 'opener of heads'. He shows him how to examine a patient and diagnose where there may be a problem in the head from an assessment of the state of consciousness and the use of the limbs. He then shows him how to remove a piece of skull and replace it with a silver plate, which is bound with bandages while they await recovery.

Although the Egyptians had accumulated this knowledge they did not recognise the importance of the brain as the organ of thought. This is understandable, since emotions often seem to relate to the chest and to the beating of the heart. During the mummification process they preserved the heart and other organs, but the brain was removed by pulling it down through the nose and discarding it. It was not believed to be needed in the afterlife.

Nevertheless, they described the state of dementia. They believed that it was related to age, although it was not something that inevitably happened to everyone.

The ancient Greeks

Hippocrates, the father of medicine, described the condition that we can recognise as dementia in the fifth century BC. Although it had been observed before then, it was considered a disorder caused by demonic possession, as in those days so many conditions were thought to have a supernatural origin. Hippocrates was one of the first doctors to suggest that the brain was the seat of the mind.

Furthermore, he differentiated between mania, melancholia and dementia. Essentially, he recognised that dementia was progressive and that it was very different from depression (melancholia) and other mental illnesses.

In the second century the Greek physician Claudius Galenus of Pergamum (AD 131–201), better known as Galen, performed several dissections on animals and accurately described many of the organs of the body. He described the function of the nerves, and examined the structures of the eyes, ears, larynx and reproductive organs. He taught that psychic gases and vital fluids called humours flowed through the body into the ventricles of the brain, thereby allowing for the development of mental functions. In his writings he also described age-related forgetfulness. This he attributed to weakening of the humours that flowed through the brain.

Aretaeus of Cappadocia at the end of the second century distinguished between acute and chronic conditions of the mind. Acute disorders, he said, were reversible and he called them delirium. Chronic disorders associated with loss of memory and other mental symptoms he called dementia. He said that these were irreversible. This, as we shall see in Chapter 8 *(Depression, delirium and mild cognitive impairment – things that can be confused with dementia)* was pretty accurate and accords with what we now know.[4]

The rise of anatomy

The early Christian Church banned the anatomical dissection of the body and it was not until the sixteenth century that further advances in knowledge about the brain were made. Andreas Vesalius (1514–1564) was a Flemish anatomist who demonstrated that Galen and other early anatomists had been incorrect in some of their conclusions. In 1543 he wrote the first anatomically accurate medical textbook, *De Humani Corporis Fabrica* (*On the Fabric of the Human Body*), complete with precise illustrations of the brain. He believed that the brain and nervous system were the seat of the mind and the emotions. Deterioration of the brain would result in diminished power of the mind.

One of King Charles I's physicians was Dr Thomas Willis (1621–1675), an anatomist who was deeply interested in the blood supply of the body. He published several books in the 1660s, the most significant being a work about the brain. In it he described the circle of blood vessels at the base of the brain, which were formed from major arteries travelling up the front of the neck to join with ones from the back of the neck to produce an arterial circle which gave off branches to supply blood to the various areas of the brain. This is called the Circle of Willis.

In 1672 he described 'dementia postapoplexy', meaning dementia arising after patients had suffered from strokes, apoplexy being the old name for stroke. He was quite correct in his conclusion, since this is one of the causes of vascular dementia, which we will look at in Chapter 5 (*Vascular dementia*).

France and the father of psychiatry

French physician Philippe Pinel (1745–1826) is regarded as the father of modern psychiatry. It was the practice before then to treat patients with mental illness in asylums and with widespread use of restraints. When he became the medical superintendent of the Hospice de la Salpêtrière in Paris, he ordered that the shackles should all be struck off the patients and he introduced humane treatments. Not only that but he began a systematic classification of mental illness and in particular started using the term 'dementia'. Although there is record of the word being used earlier, this was the first instance of its use as a medical diagnosis.

At about the same time another French physician, Jean-Étienne Esquirol (1772–1840), wrote a book called *Des Maladies Mentales* in which he listed a range of causes of dementia, including those we would recognise today, such as repeated head injuries and mercury poisoning, but also fanciful causes like haemorrhoids, masturbation and domestic problems. Nevertheless, it was an attempt to search for reasons why people might have developed the condition.

Pathology and Alzheimer's disease

In the nineteenth century, post-mortem anatomical examination became an accepted part of medical science. It allowed doctors to examine organs and correlate pathological changes with signs and symptoms experienced by patients in life, in order to build up a real picture of what happens in disease.

Arnold Pick, a Czech physician (1851–1924), was professor of neurology and psychiatry at Prague. In 1892 he described a condition in which there is atrophy of the frontal and temporal lobes of the brain (see Chapter 2), which resulted in senile dementia. It became known as Pick's lobar atrophy, one of the rarer types of dementia. He went on to write a book on neuropathology.

Emil Kraepelin (1856–1926) was a German psychiatrist, now regarded as the founder of scientific psychiatry. He believed that most mental disorders had a biological basis and that this could be defined in pathological changes that could be found in the brain. He did important work with many of the severe mental disorders, including bipolar disorder and schizophrenia.

A colleague of his was Alois Alzheimer (1864–1915), a German psychiatrist and neuropathologist. When he was working in the Frankfurt Asylum in 1901, he observed a 51-year-old female patient with significant memory and behavioural problems. When she died he examined her brain using staining techniques. These showed the presence of amyloid plaques and neurofibrillary tangles. He thereby described for the first time the pathological signs of dementia (see Chapter 4, *Alzheimer's disease*).

Kraepelin wrote a textbook subsequent to Alzheimer's discovery in which he referred to two types of dementia: a presenile variant which he called Alzheimer's disease and a senile type. This differentiation into two types was maintained in the textbooks for decades, until it was realised that they were not two separate conditions and that age was not a valid differentiator; the pathological changes were the same. Nevertheless, as we shall see later, it is important to consider the needs of what we now call early-onset dementia.

Otto Binswanger (1852–1929) was a Swiss psychiatrist and neurologist who also did extensive work on the brain. In 1894 he described a condition which he called 'encephalitis subcorticalis chronica progressiva', which was associated with memory problems and intellectual difficulties. It is one of the rare forms of dementia and is due to small blood vessel damage to the white matter of the brain. Today we know it as subcortical dementia or Binswanger's disease (see Chapter 5, *Vascular dementia*).

Dementia around the world

Dementia is not something that people like to think about – not just individuals, but society as a whole. It is, in fact, a colossal problem throughout the world, as the following figures show:

KEY POINTS

- Globally, there are more than 35.6 million people with one or other form of dementia.
- Globally there are 7.7 million new cases every year.
- In the European Union there are currently 5 million people with dementia.
- Dementia is not a disease only of developed countries – 60 per cent of cases of dementia occur in developing countries.
- Between 2 and 5 per cent of new cases start before the age of 65 years.
- In 2012 the global estimated cost of dementia was $604 billion.

In 2012 the World Health Organisation produced a report, Dementia – a Public Health Priority. It set out a fairly stark picture, suggesting that the world faces a dementia time bomb. It acknowledges that people are living longer and that there have been significant improvements in health, especially through vaccination and better management of infectious diseases. On the other hand, the incidence of non-communicable disease, including dementia, is increasing. In part the rise in the number of cases of dementia is because of this increase in life expectancy.

The report suggests that because people go on living for many years after the diagnosis of dementia, it is imperative that adequate support should be available for people living with the disease.

The UK situation

The UK has a population of over 63 million, the third largest in the European Union.[5] According to Alzheimer's Society, in 2013 there were more than 800,000 people with dementia in the UK, comprising:

- More than 665,000 in England

- More than 86,000 in Scotland

- More than 18,000 in Northern Ireland

- More than 44,000 in Wales.

There are 163,000 new cases of dementia in the UK every year.

In the UK about 25 million people, or 42 per cent of the population, know a close friend or relative with dementia (Alzheimer's Research UK). Dementia is commoner in older people, but it occurs in all ages:

- One in 1,400 people aged 40–64 years have dementia.

- One in 100 people aged 65–69 years have dementia.

- One in 25 people aged 70–79 years have dementia.

- One in 6 people aged 80 years and over have dementia.

In 2013 dementia was recorded as the 3rd most common cause of death in the UK, after heart disease and stroke.

Early onset dementia

Early onset dementia is when dementia occurs in people under the age of 65 years. It may also be called dementia in younger people or young-age dementia. Currently, there are more than 44,000 people in the UK with early onset dementia.

The symptoms experienced can be exactly the same as with any other form of the condition, but the needs of the person with early onset dementia may be different.

For example, a person with early onset dementia may:

- Be in employment

- Have a partner who is in employment

- Have children dependent on him or her

- Have parents who may be dependent on him or her

- Have financial commitments.

The cause of early onset dementia can be the same as with dementia affecting people over the age of 65 years. Alzheimer's disease is still the commonest cause, but it makes up only a third of cases, whereas in older people it makes up two thirds. Vascular dementia is the next most common, causing 20 per cent of cases. However, fronto-temporal dementia causes 12 per cent of early onset dementia compared to only 2 per cent of cases in older people.

Diagnosis in this group is often delayed, partly because it is often not considered at a younger age and because the person may not ask for help or even realise that they have a problem. Once dementia is suspected, the GP will usually refer their patient to a neurologist rather than to a psychiatrist, because of the need to pinpoint the diagnosis.

KEY POINTS

- Globally, two thirds of people with dementia are female.
- Globally, one in three people over the age of 65 years will develop dementia before they die.
- In the UK only 43 per cent of people with dementia have a diagnosis.

Future prospects

The World Health Organisation estimates that the number of people around the world living with dementia will double by 2030 and triple by 2050. There is one new case of dementia every four seconds.

According to Alzheimer's Society the number of people with dementia in the UK will rise dramatically as the population ages. It is estimated that whereas in 2014 there were 800,000 people with dementia in the UK, this figure will rise to one million by 2021 and to 1.7 million by 2051.

FAMOUS PEOPLE WHO HAVE HAD OR HAVE DEMENTIA

There is no shame in having dementia. Everyone can leave their own mark in life and this should be celebrated. We should strive to help every person with dementia to live well. All of these people had or have dementia yet all have contributed to the world:

- Ronald Reagan (1911–2004), film actor and 40th President of the USA – diagnosed with Alzheimer's disease in 1994.

- Charles Bronson (1921–2003), film actor noted for his tough guy roles.

- Rita Hayworth (1918–1987), film actor – diagnosed with Alzheimer's disease in 1980.

- Iris Murdoch (1919–1999), award-winning writer – diagnosed with Alzheimer's disease in 1997.

- Otto Preminger (1905–1986), Austrian theatre and film director.

- Ferenc Puskás (1927–2006), legendary Hungarian footballer.

- Sir Terry Pratchett (born 1948), English author of the Discworld series, announced in 2007 that he was suffering from early onset dementia, specifically posterior subcortical atrophy.

Chapter 2

Understand the brain

The brain is the most important organ in the body. It controls the way that you move, and it perceives all of the information that is transmitted to it from the sense organs of touch, vision, hearing, smell and taste. It is also where you perceive pain.

You might say that the brain is the essence of the individual, since it is where all of the thinking and emotions seem to take place. That is, the brain seems to be the seat of the mind, an idea widely debated by philosophers and scientists almost since the beginning of human consciousness. We will come back to this later in the chapter, since it is important in our understanding of the brain and our consideration of dementia.

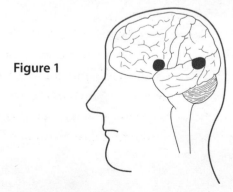

Figure 1

BASIC BRAIN FACTS:

- The average adult brain weighs about three pounds.
- The brain has a texture like firm jelly.
- The brain is made up of about one hundred billion cells.
- About a quarter of the blood pumped out by the heart with every heartbeat goes to supply the brain.
- The brain uses about 20 per cent of the body's oxygen.
- The brain needs a continuous supply of oxygen. A few minutes of oxygen deprivation will lead to irreversible damage.
- The brain looks wrinkled and not unlike a walnut. Those wrinkles are called convolutions and are where you do your thinking.

The nervous system

The nervous system is the body's main communication system. It is customary to consider it as having two parts, the central nervous system, consisting of the brain and spinal cord, and the peripheral nervous system, consisting of the nerves to the various parts of the body. In addition, there is the autonomic nervous system, which controls the function of the internal organs.

The nervous system controls every aspect of your life, ranging from the involuntary functions like breathing to the voluntary functions of moving. The brain, of course, is the great computer of the body where all the information from sensory nerves is transmitted and where thoughts and decisions are made, and it is from there that nerve impulses are transmitted down motor nerves to make muscles move.

The nineteenth century – major advances

The Victorian era saw an explosion in knowledge in all areas of science, including medicine. In regard to the brain there were three major discoveries.

The speech centre

In the mid-nineteenth century the French surgeon and anthropologist Pierre Paul Broca (1824–1880) discovered that the left hemisphere of the brain was dominant in speech production. He localised this to a very specific area in the frontal lobe of the dominant hemisphere. It was named after him as Broca's area.

Language comprehension

Not long after Broca's discovery, Carl Wernicke (1848–1905), a German anatomist and psychiatrist, discovered another area of the brain associated with the way we understand language and writing. This also was found in the dominant hemisphere, but is towards the back of the temporal area. It is known as Wernicke's area.

Memory

The Russian psychiatrist Sergei Korsakoff (1854–1900) studied the effects of alcoholism. He found that in advanced cases patients became paranoid, developed memory problems and could eventually manifest a type of movement disorder or stagger that is called ataxia. From anatomical examination of the brains of people with such problems he found that they had developed a specific nutritional deficiency (later found to be vitamin B1 or thiamine), which caused structural changes in areas in the middle of the brain. He deduced that these areas were associated with the ability to remember. As a result, we now know that the temporal lobes of the brain are associated with memory function.

The all-important nerve cells

The nervous system is made up of two basic types of cells, neurones and glial cells. Neurones transmit information from cell to cell. Glial cells do not transmit information but provide structure and form to nerves and the brain.

Neurones

These are the basic functional cells of the nervous system. There are actually many different types of neurones, which come in different shapes and sizes depending on where they are situated in the nervous system, since this has a bearing on what they are needed to do.

Their basic structure consists of a body (called a soma), an axon and dendrites. The axon carries information away from the body or soma, whereas the dendrites, which are wispy, tentacle-like projections, receive information and convey it to the body.

The axons produce a protein called tau, which is essential for maintaining the shape of the neurone. As we shall see later, excessive and abnormal tau may be produced in Alzheimer's disease.

The axon is coated in a myelin sheath, which acts rather like the insulating coating of an electrical wire, to stop electrical impulses being discharged too early. In the condition of multiple sclerosis the myelin sheaths degenerate, so nerve impulses are not transmitted down nerves, resulting in various degrees of malfunction of the nervous system and eventually paralysis.

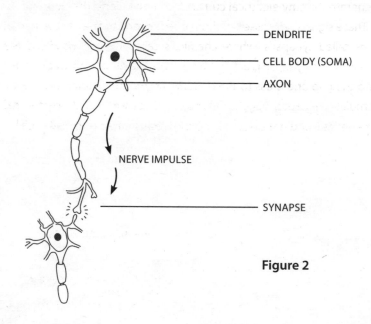

Figure 2

Myelin sheaths give nerves a white appearance, which we will consider in the section on white matter that follows.

The neurone works by transmitting messages as electrical signals known as nerve impulses. They do this by an electrochemical process.

Chemicals in the body are electrically charged, depending on whether they have lost or gained electrons. They are called ions. In the nervous system the most important ions are sodium and potassium, which both have a single positive charge, and calcium, which has a double positive charge, and chloride, which has a single negative charge.

An impulse is sent down the axon by a process called the action potential. Fluctuations between the ions in and out of the cell generate this tiny electrical current that flows along the neurone.

These signals are passed on from one neurone to the next at special sites called synapses, where chemicals called neurotransmitters are released. The synapse is actually a tiny gap. The neurotransmitters flow into the gap and cross to the dendrite on the other side, where they stimulate a receptor site, the result being that a further action potential is generated and the electrical impulse is transmitted from cell to cell.

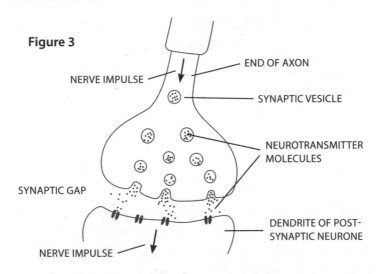

Figure 3

NERVE IMPULSE

END OF AXON

SYNAPTIC VESICLE

NEUROTRANSMITTER MOLECULES

SYNAPTIC GAP

DENDRITE OF POST-SYNAPTIC NEURONE

NERVE IMPULSE

The human brain has about 100 billion neurones. They are incredibly complex and each cell will make connections with thousands of other neurones. Thus there are trillions of connections within the system.

Glial cells

There are about ten times as many glial cells as there are neurones. There are various types (astrocytes, oligodendrocytes, microglia and

Schwann cells), each of which has a different function. Basically, they provide support to the neurones, supply them with nutrients and have a defensive function.

White matter and grey matter

If you enjoy the crime fiction of Agatha Christie then you may well have heard her detective Hercule Poirot saying, that 'it is a case for the little grey cells'. He is referring to the thinking part of the brain, the grey cells that compose the grey matter.

The outer part or the surface of the brain, called the cortex, has a greyish-pink appearance due to the type of nerve cells that it contains. These are the bodies of the neurones. They have no covering of myelin, hence their grey-pink appearance. This is where the dendrites and most of the synapses are found. The cerebral cortex and most of the cerebellum consists of grey matter, as does the central core of the spinal cord.

The deeper tissue of the brain and cerebellum, called the medulla, and the outer part of the spinal cord and the peripheral nerves are made up of myelinated nerve fibres. As mentioned earlier, this makes them appear white. Because these make up the deeper tissue of the brain and the outer surface of nerves, they are called white matter. Essentially, this is the conducting tissue, or the wiring part of the nervous system.

Neurotransmitters

There are half a dozen major neurotransmitters involved in different parts of the nervous system.

Acetylcholine

This is the main neurotransmitter within the cholinergic pathways, which are the main pathways in the brainstem. These are associated with cognitive functions and mainly with memory. It is thought that disruption of these pathways is the probable cause of Alzheimer's disease.

Outside the brain acetylcholine is the main neurotransmitter of the parasympathetic nervous system.

Dopamine

This monoamine neurotransmitter is mainly involved in the parts of the brain called the basal ganglia, which are responsible for making our movements smooth, rather than rigid and robotic. Dopamine is also involved in cognition and in feelings of pleasure.

A deficiency of dopamine contributes to Parkinson's disease, while an excess is thought to play a part in the development of schizophrenia. As we shall see in Chapter 6, it may have relevance in dementia in respect to Lewy bodies.

Noradrenaline

This is a monoamine neurotransmitter. It is involved in attention, arousal and pleasure feelings.

Outside the brain it is the main transmitter of the sympathetic nervous system.

Serotonin

This has the reputation of being the happiness neurotransmitter. It controls mood and appetite, and may be involved in sleep control.

Serotonin is one of the main neurotransmitters in the body. Its proper name is 5-hydroxytryptamine or 5-HT. It is a monoamine neurotransmitter, which is mainly built up from the amino acid tryptophan.

Only 20 per cent of the serotonin in the body is found in the brain and nervous system. The majority is found in certain cells in the gut, where its function is to regulate the way that the bowel moves.

People who are depressed may have lower levels in the brain. For these patients we commonly use a group of antidepressant drugs called the selective serotonin reuptake inhibitors, the SSRIs, which keep the levels of serotonin topped up so that brain cells function better and communicate with each other, and mood is lifted.

Glutamate

This is the main excitatory neurotransmitter in the brain. This means that it is involved in many of the functions of the brain, including memory, thinking and learning.

Gamma-Aminobutyric acid (GABA)

This by contrast is an inhibitory neurotransmitter. It reduces activity. It is used by about half the cells in the brain.

The parts of the brain

We are now in a position to have a look at the different parts of the brain in order to see which parts control which aspects of our body functions.

The brain has two halves, a right side and a left side. Each side is divided into lobes, which have different functions.

The outer surface of the brain is called the cortex. It consists of grey matter. The deeper tissue of the brain is called the medulla. It is made of white matter.

The basic brain structures are known as the following in medicine:

- The cerebrum, consisting of the two cerebral hemispheres
- The brainstem
- The cerebellum, consisting of two cerebellar hemispheres.

The cerebrum

This makes up two thirds of the whole brain and is where we think, perceive, create and plan. It is where we organise thoughts to produce language, solve problems, philosophise and experience life.

All this varied activity takes place in the cerebral cortex, the outer surface of grey matter which contains all of the neurones, dendrites and synapses and is also where we perceive all the information from our sense organs and control our body movements.

The cerebrum is made up of a right hemisphere and a left hemisphere. The right hemisphere controls the left side of the body and the left hemisphere controls the right side of the body.

Each cerebral hemisphere has four lobes.

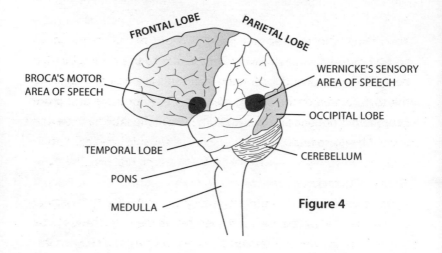

Figure 4

- The frontal lobe is where reasoning, calculation, problem solving and judgement take place. Broca's area, which controls speech, is usually in the frontal lobe.

- The parietal lobe is where pain and touch are processed.

- The temporal lobe, which is mainly concerned with memory, is also associated with emotions and speech. Wernicke's area, which controls language recognition, is located in the temporal lobe in the left hemisphere. Sound is also perceived in the temporal lobes.

- The occipital lobe, at the back of the brain, is associated with the perception of vision. This may be the most surprising finding, since one would expect vision to be perceived near to the eyes, but in fact the pathways involved are quite complex.

The brain's wrinkled appearance on account of numerous ridges and furrows, known as convolutions, is due to the cerebral cortex being folded back and forth upon itself. This is a way of increasing the surface area of the cortex, creating space for more and more neurones without having to expand the size of the skull. Each crevice formed by these folds is called a sulcus (plural, sulci) and each ridge or fold between the crevices is called a gyrus (plural, gyri). There are about thirty of these.

Most people have a **dominant hemisphere**, which in the majority of right-handed people means the left hemisphere. This tends to be the hemisphere which contains the speech centres, so if such a right-handed person has a left hemisphere stroke they will experience speech problems and will have right-side-of-body paralysis and sensory loss.

From this evidence you would imagine that, similarly, the majority of naturally left-handed people would have a dominant right hemisphere. This is not always the case. About fifty per cent have dominance of the right and fifty per cent have dominance of the left hemisphere.

Certain functions of the mind seem to be associated with either the right or left hemisphere of the brain. This has become known as the right brain vs. left brain theory of mind, and is based on the work of psychobiologist Robert Sperry (1913–1994), for which in 1981 he received a Nobel Prize.

Sperry's work has given us some very good insight into the brain–mind connection and delineated functions that seem more associated with one hemisphere than the other. It does not mean that they are exclusively associated in that way, for other work indicates that in many ways the brain is holographic, in that all parts of the brain have the potential to operate the mind, so that if there is injury to the organ other parts may be able to take over lost function. So it is more a case of pre-eminence of associations rather than exclusive association.

RIGHT HEMISPHERE	LEFT HEMISPHERE
Visual	Verbal
Intuitive	Logical
Creative	Analytical
Artistic	Scientific
Musical	Mathematical
Pattern recognition – see pictures	Item recognition – see links
Lateral thinking	Linear thinking
Emotions	Clinical
Physically expressive	Verbally expressive
Hears nuances	Hears sounds
Poor time sense or awareness	Good time sense and awareness
Poor organisation	Good organisation

Table 1 Right and left hemisphere associations

Some people seem to be more one-sided than the other; in other words, their brains and minds seem to operate with one prominent hemisphere, so that we talk about right hemisphere dominance or left hemisphere dominance. It is important to appreciate that this does not mean that only one side works, but that the functions of one side seem to be most to the fore in the way that they think and live.

The two hemispheres are connected by a part of the brain called the corpus callosum. It is a bridge where nerve pathways pass over from one hemisphere to the other side of the body. This results in the left side of the brain controlling the right side of the body, and the right hemisphere controlling the left side of the body.

The ventricles

Within the brain substance there is a network of four cavities filled with cerebrospinal fluid. These link up with the central canal of the spinal cord, and their function is to bathe and cushion the brain and spinal cord. The cerebrospinal fluid also has a role in bringing nutrients to the brain and removing waste products from it.

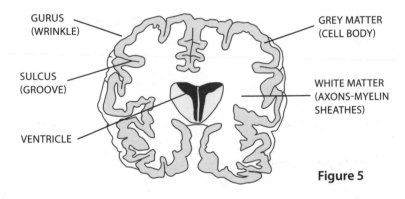

Figure 5

The brainstem

This is the part of the brain that is made up of the midbrain, pons and medulla. It basically controls all the vital life functions, such as heartbeat, blood pressure and breathing.

Midbrain

Within the brainstem the midbrain is the part that controls emotions and stores memories. Nowadays we mainly refer to it as the 'limbic system'. It is actually found on the inner surface of each cerebral hemisphere and forms a circuit around the ventricles. Thus the limbic system has two halves, like the other structures of the brain.

The limbic system consists of the following structures:

- The amygdala, an almond-shaped structure (its name being the Latin for almond), which has a role in storing deep emotional memories. It seems to control fear and is responsible for activating all the unpleasant sensations we experience when frightened, such as palpitations, butterflies in the stomach, sweaty hands and shivers. There is also mounting evidence that it is associated with addictive tendencies.

- The hippocampus, which is involved in memory storing and memory processing. It is shaped a little like a seahorse, hence its name, which comes from the Greek.

- The hypothalamus, the workhorse of the brain, regulating many of our internal functions, such as thirst, appetite, sleep cycle and internal balance of metabolism, temperature control and circadian rhythms.

- The thalamus, the great signal box of the brain. It relays information from all of the sense organs to the higher parts of the brain where the information is processed and the experiences of the senses are perceived. It has a large part to play in pain perception as well as being the relay centre for movements.

The pons

This is a bridge-like structure connecting the lobes of the midbrain, medulla and cerebrum. It is derived from the Latin for bridge and is known as the *pons Varolii* (the bridge of Varolio) after Costanzo Varolio (1543–1575), the Italian anatomist who discovered it. Its function is to regulate sleep and it controls one's level of consciousness.

The medulla oblongata

This is the lowermost part of the brainstem. It controls all the autonomic functions of the body, meaning the involuntary functions like the heartbeat, breathing and digestion.

The medulla oblongata connects directly with the spinal cord, which relays information to and from the brain to the rest of the body.

Thus the brainstem is the part of the brain that takes care of our basic life functions, such as control of our heartbeat and breathing, and is also our instinctive brain, controlling our survival instincts, our sexual desires and our basic needs.

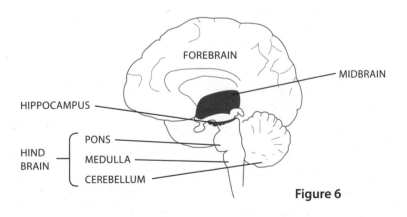

Figure 6

The cerebellum

The cerebellum is the large structure at the back and the bottom of the brain, which controls the coordination of movement and balance. It has a right and a left hemisphere, like a miniature cerebrum. Its surface is covered in grey matter.

The cranial nerves

There are twelve pairs of special nerves that emerge directly from the brain. Some of these nerves have a sensory function and carry information from the eyes, ears, nose and mouth. Others have a motor function and send messages from the brain to control the muscles of the head and throat. Others supply various glands or important organs like the heart and lungs.

The spinal nerves

These are nerves that emerge from the spinal cord and pass through gaps in the vertebral column to supply the trunk and limbs.

The autonomic nervous system

This is another important part of the nervous system, separate from the central nervous system (brain and spinal cord and peripheral nerves). It controls many of the involuntary functions of the body.

There are two main components to it:

- Sympathetic nervous system – which prepares us for fight or flight.

- Parasympathetic nervous system – which controls the functions that allow us to rest and digest.

The sympathetic and parasympathetic systems by and large produce opposite yet complementary effects. You can think of the sympathetic nervous system's role as preparing your body for an emergency, while the parasympathetic nervous system restores normal functioning after the emergency has passed.

The mind and the brain

Most people feel that their personality, their consciousness – all those things that the individual recognises as their own self – is located in their head. It is as if the individual is inside the head, looking out at the world beyond.

Psychologists and neurobiologists are nowadays fortunate in having two very effective types of scanners, called functional Magnetic Resonance Imaging (fMRI) and Positive Emission Tomography (PET). These allow researchers to virtually picture what is happening inside the brain during certain activities or when someone is thinking different types of thought.

Although it is something of an oversimplification, we can basically say that the functions of the mind mirror the anatomy of the brain that we have so far considered.

- The rational mind is associated with the functioning of the frontal lobes. It seems to have much to do with the development and expression of our personality.

- Creativity and artistic ability seem to be right hemisphere functions of the mind.

- Logic and mathematical ability seem to be left hemisphere functions of the mind.

- Our emotional mind seems to be associated with the limbic system or the midbrain.

- Our instinctive mind processes seem to be associated with the brainstem.

We are now in a position to consider what happens during dementia in the next chapter.

Chapter 3

What happens in dementia

It is very important to understand that dementia is an umbrella label, in the same way that arthritis refers to a number of different conditions affecting the joints. The differing pathologies can produce different clinical pictures, which we shall consider when we look at them individually. They do all, however, have enough common features to allow us to give an overview of what happens.

The ageing brain

Dementia is not a normal part of ageing. It is the name for a group of conditions that cause damage to the brain. Before we begin, I want to describe what happens to the brain as we age normally.

Like all organs of the body, the brain loses mass and cells and its function tends to deteriorate as we age. The shrinkage of the brain starts at about the age of 50 years. This is mainly the result of water loss. From the age of 50 to 65 years the average brain may lose 4 or 5 ounces in weight.

The effect of this is to cause widening of the sulci, the folds of the cortex, and in the ventricles within the brain. This can be shown on Magnetic Resonance Imaging (MRI), one of the tests used to diagnose dementia, which we shall consider in Chapter 9 (*Getting the ball rolling*).

The loss of cells in the brain with normal ageing is less than was once believed, with recent studies showing selective neuronal loss from a few specific areas as opposed to a more generalised loss. The level of neurotransmitters also tends to drop, which seems to explain the loss of some of our cognitive functions as we get older. Moreover, the brain's ability to absorb glucose, which it needs to function, is also reduced.

At the functional level, people may experience a slowing down of their mental abilities. People often notice that they can't do things as quickly as they used to, which may be the result of a reduction in the overall number of synapses, the connections between nerve cells. Effectively, the circuit board of memory and of mental functioning just has fewer connections. The difference between this normal aspect of ageing and dementia is that in normal ageing the abilities are retained but just slow down, whereas in dementia the abilities are gradually lost.

Memory difficulty is something that worries a lot of people as they enter middle age. Slight difficulty remembering names or experiencing the 'tip of the tongue' phenomenon, when they cannot quite bring a word or name to mind no matter how hard they try, often makes them worry that they are starting to develop dementia. This is actually incredibly common and in most cases does not mean that the person concerned is developing dementia.

Indeed, there is a state that is called mild cognitive impairment in which this is common, but again it is not the same as dementia. We shall consider it in Chapter 8 (*Depression, delirium and mild cognitive impairment – things that can be confused with dementia*).

KEY POINTS

- Dementia is the name for a group of symptoms that occur when the brain is damaged by very specific diseases.
- Dementia is commoner with increasing age but is not the result of increasing age.

Common symptoms of dementia

So far we have considered the normal changes that occur with age. Now we are going to consider what sort of symptoms occur in the conditions that cause dementia. These occur on top of normal ageing and are far more extreme and not simply an exaggeration of normal ageing.

Dementia may present in different ways. The following symptoms will tend to manifest at some stage:

- Memory difficulty

- Communication problems

- Difficulty in understanding

- Disorientation

- Reduced ability to concentrate

- Emotional changes

- Behaviour changes

- Loneliness

- Personality change.

49

Memory problems

The characteristic problem that tends to happen in dementia is that the memory for recent events, the short-term memory, starts to deteriorate. By contrast, the long-term memory remains intact, so that the person can recall events from twenty to fifty years ago as if they had just occurred.

In dementia names, dates and places may be forgotten. As it progresses, the number and type of things that cannot be remembered may increase. For example, PIN numbers, telephone numbers and addresses may be forgotten. So too with often travelled paths, so that the person forgets how to get somewhere they used to go regularly.

Difficulty with communication

A person with dementia may start to lose their vocabulary. They may retreat from conversations with family and friends because they find it difficult to converse. They may lose their grasp of a discussion and feel unable to formulate their thoughts.

Communication is not merely to do with the spoken voice, but also body language, facial expressions, smiling and even physical contact. In dementia, the parts of the brain that deal with these things become affected. The temporal lobes, which deal with language understanding, are commonly affected, as are the frontal lobes, which are concerned with behaviour.

The person with dementia may therefore start to become isolated, because they find it increasingly difficult to communicate. They can feel pressured to communicate and may feel distressed as a result, leading them to withdraw in order to avoid that distress. People around them may feel that they are deliberately isolating themselves, yet it is all a result of an underlying brain disease that is causing dementia.

Difficulty in understanding

We take so many things for granted once we have learned to do them. Driving, playing an instrument, doing any number of complex tasks – we learn them and then repetition makes them second nature. In dementia there may seem to be an unlearning taking place. Complex tasks may prove difficult as the person fails to understand why a certain step in the process is needed. As the condition worsens, even simpler things may seem beyond the person's understanding. For instance, they may not understand how to switch on a light, unlock a door or boil an egg. Putting milk in the oven or a meal in the fridge instead of the oven, or putting shopping in the wrong cupboard, may all be examples that the person is no longer understanding the process.

They may also not understand that certain things are dangerous. In advanced dementia this can prove dangerous not only to the individual but also to the carers if the person with dementia tries to light a fire by burning newspapers, or lift hot objects like pans of boiling water.

Disorientation

People with dementia can lose sense of time, place and person as the condition progresses. They can lose track of the day, the date, the month and even the year. Indeed, in the advanced stages they can believe that they are living at a different time, that their own long-dead parents are still with them, or that they are the brother or sister of their own children.

They can get disorientated by place, so that they are confused about where they are. This can lead them to wander away from their home at odd times of the day or night, sometimes getting lost. They can ultimately get disorientated about who they are and, if found wandering, may not remember their name or where they live.

Reduced ability to concentrate

It is common for people to stop doing long-cherished hobbies that demand concentration, since they may find it hard to focus or concentrate on the activity. Their attention span may drop continuously to the point where they are not able to focus on anything for longer than a few minutes.

People with dementia give up reading and doing crosswords, Sudoku or puzzles. They may stop knitting, playing games, gardening, housecleaning or cooking.

Emotional changes

All kinds of emotional change can occur. Some people may become weepy and tearful when they were previously stoical. Others may become irritable or have temper tantrums, when they were previously placid. Yet others may start to develop unpredictable mood swings. Indeed, depression and anxiety are both common and need to be addressed, because someone who is suffering from dementia may improve markedly if their depression is treated. It can often be missed, because the intense lowness of mood that is characteristic of depression at other ages is not always present.

Some people develop emotional lability. This means that their emotions may change rapidly, without obvious cause, or they may react to a situation with excess emotion. Thus they may weep continuously, yet not know why they are doing so; this may or may not be because they are depressed. Or they may become irritable, vexed or angry in a manner that is out of proportion to a given situation.

Behavioural changes

Dementia can be a frightening process for people. They can feel anxious, depressed, angry, isolated and frustrated.

Sometimes they show the loop phenomenon, in which it seems they get stuck in a thought they cannot get out of, instead repeating the same question over and over again. Even if an answer is given, it simply does not register, so the loop continues, the cycle being replayed to the frustration of carer or family, who may be asked where someone is six times in as many minutes, the person with dementia having forgotten the answer that was given on each occasion.

This can happen to an action as well, resulting in repetitive pacing or repetitive, purposeless movements. Such activity is not done for exercise, but simply walking and pacing because the person feels driven to do so. In the later stages of the disease this can take the form of wandering around the home at any time of the day or night, or even wandering away from the home and getting lost.

Inappropriate behaviour can also occur. The person may shout, scream or become aggressive, while suspiciousness is common. The person with dementia may start to think that people are watching them or that people are stealing from them or talking about them when they are not watching.

Neglect of the self is common. It can begin with a loss of interest in their appearance, so that they can start to look unkempt, before progressing to the point where they stop washing, shaving or brushing their hair. In advanced stages, they may lose any sense of propriety, to the point where they inadvertently expose themselves, urinate in public and so on. Similarly, they may lose inhibitions about sex, touching and caressing people inappropriately. Again, this can be highly embarrassing for carers and family.

These are all potential behavioural changes that may occur.

Loneliness

I mentioned earlier that people with dementia can become isolated. It might be that they withdraw, but they may also become isolated. And if they do become isolated, they can easily become lonely.

Currently about a third of people with dementia live on their own, and many experience feelings of loneliness.

- 24 per cent of people in general over the age of 55 feel lonely.

- 38 per cent of people over the age of 55 with dementia feel lonely.

- 62 per cent of people with dementia who live on their own feel lonely.

Personality change

This is something that may seem to happen relatively quickly, or it can take a long time and only slowly creep over the person. It can be quite harrowing for family and friends to see the personality of their loved one change so drastically. Their way of thinking, their way of behaving and their recognition of others may seem to drift away, until the person that they once were seems very different from the person they have now become.

Yet it is important to remember that it is, after all, the same person. The alteration in their personality is not deliberate, not contrived, but comes about through brain damage from a progressive disease. There is still good reason to nurture and love the person for all of their qualities.

Getting a diagnosis

If you or someone close to you seems to be experiencing any of the above symptoms, then it is important to see your GP in order to have some tests done to see whether dementia could be the problem.

Let's look again at some of the statistics. Firstly, only 43 per cent of people with dementia have had a diagnosis made. Secondly, about a third of people with dementia live on their own. This implies that many people with dementia are soldiering on, not necessarily coping well, and receiving less care than most people would expect them to receive. This is made worse by the fact that 62 per cent of people with dementia who are living on their own feel lonely – almost double the figure found in people who live alone but do not have dementia. So these people are not living well with their dementia. This is why it is vital to get a diagnosis in order to start putting supports in place.

What happens to the brain in dementia?

All of the symptoms we have just considered come about as the result of damage to the brain. How quickly changes occur depends upon what is causing them, which condition is producing the damage and which areas of the brain are being affected. Some types are slowly progressive, while others are quite rapid.

Essentially, in dementia brain cells die off faster than they normally would. The more brain cells that die, the less able the brain is to function. Tasks that previously could be performed will be performed less well, and the cognitive ability of the individual will tend to deteriorate, so that attention, understanding and problem solving will diminish.

If parts of the brain that deal with emotion are damaged then this will produce emotional changes. If parts of the brain that deal with behaviour, mainly the frontal parts of the brain, are damaged then there are likely to be personality and behavioural changes.

Depending upon which condition is causing the problem, there will be different effects on the brain substance, and there may be differing effects on the various neurotransmitters. This is why getting the right diagnosis is so important, because different treatments may be indicated. We will be looking at this in later chapters.

The basic effect of all dementias is to produce:

- Premature loss of brain cells through their premature death

- Shrinking of the brain

- Destruction of the cortex with deterioration in intellect and memory, and alteration of emotions and behaviour.

KEY POINTS

- Dementia is a progressive disease that causes deterioration of brain function.

- Different causes of dementia (different diseases) produce different patterns of dementia.
- Specific diagnosis is important because different diseases may need different treatment.

Why short-term memory goes but the past is remembered

This is something that puzzles most carers of people with dementia. The loss of short-term memory becomes very apparent, as the person forgets recent events or even things that have just happened, yet can talk about things from their past, even their childhood, with absolute clarity.

This is one of the things that can often delay the person or their family from seeking help, because they are reassured by the long-term memory preservation. The impression is that if they can remember things from the distant past, then there can't be too much wrong with the memory. And the short-term loss is just attributed to getting older.

This apparent disparity comes about because of the way that memory is stored. When something happens that is committed to memory, it gets imprinted on the neural circuits of cells. We call this process 'imprinting'. Thus the longer a memory is there, the more it gets reinforced and imprinted, so that long-term memories are effectively etched into the memory bank.

Short-term memories by definition have not been reinforced and are not fully imprinted. When brain cells die off, the most recent memories are lost because they are in the cells that die off first. So the capacity of the person with dementia to retain new memory is lost. It is rather like saving memories to the hard drive of the computer; once saved, they are retained. Short-term memories are like temporary files; a computer crash can result in the loss of all the temporary files and the information that was in them.

> **KEY POINTS**
>
> - Just because the person can remember things from long ago does not mean their memory is not affected.
> - Loss of short-term memory may be significant and should be tested by your doctor.

The stages of dementia

We can broadly divide the progression of dementia into three stages. Having said this, it is also important to understand that the course of the condition varies from person to person, even where the cause in a given group of people is the same condition. Thus five people with Alzheimer's disease may exhibit five different clusters of symptoms, though probably all with some degree of similarity. Moreover, their condition may progress at five different rates.

Early stage

This usually begins with slight changes that may be observed by the person or by those close to him or her. This might be a change in memory, or a change in their ability to do tasks that they normally did without any problem, or it could be a change of behaviour.

Sometimes the onset may be missed, because it seems to have been provoked by a life event, such as the bereavement of a partner or relative. Or it may simply be attributed to ageing.

Any of the following may be seen:

- Short-term memory problems such as forgetting messages, conversations or events

- A tendency to repeat themselves

- Failing to understand something that they would previously have grasped

- Becoming easily confused

- Having difficulty finding words

- Becoming increasingly indecisive or making errors of judgement

- Losing interest in their hobbies

- Increasing suspiciousness

- Irritability and a tendency to blame others for things that can't be found

- Starting to withdraw from social gatherings.

There is a great need to identify this stage and to put in as much support as possible. This does not mean doing everything or arranging to have everything done for them; rather the opposite, since the person needs to stay orientated, feel valued and feel able to maintain their independence. Maintaining ego and self-worth are extremely important.

You can live well and enjoy life in the early stage, which may go on for several years. There may also be drugs that will help, and the sooner they are given (if appropriate for the person and the type of dementia that they have), the more likely they are to help alleviate some of the symptoms.

We shall be looking at this in more detail later in the book, when we come to its second part, on dealing with dementia.

Middle stage

This is where all the things in stage one become more apparent. They will start to become more disabling and it may be that the person is less able to deal with day-to-day tasks. They may not remember to eat or drink, or they may forget whether or not they have had medication or meals. They may become disorientated about the time, so that they get up at inappropriate hours, thinking that night is morning and vice versa. As well as forgetfulness, at this stage the loop phenomenon will become more obvious than before.

They may start to show behavioural changes. This may include a change in personality, becoming paranoid or suspicious, becoming aggressive, or becoming shy and apathetic. They may seem disinhibited and stop looking after their appearance. They may appear unkempt or dress inappropriately – for example, mistaking underpants for a scarf, putting underclothes on top of other clothes, or putting things on back to front.

However, this is still a time when you can live well with dementia. This stage can also go on for several years.

DISINHIBITIONS

This is the name for the loss of control of one's impulses. In childhood we learn how to control urges. That is, we develop inhibitions that stop us from doing things that are inappropriate in society. Thus, you do not reach out and caress a stranger, touch your own genitals or spit in public. Similarly, you do not swear at people or say things that are offensive.

In dementia these inhibitions that stop us doing these things are lost, hence *disinhibition*. Someone with dementia may do any of these inappropriate things, because the parts of their brains that stop them are no longer working.

It is not something that you should judge someone for. They cannot help it. What you can do is learn how to deal with their behaviour, though not in a punitive manner.

Late stage

By this point the person with dementia will need help and will probably need constant nursing care. Their memory may be so poor that they do not recognise friends, family or even their spouse. Their emotions may be blunted or can be exaggerated.

Their ability to communicate may become so impaired that they cannot speak. Nevertheless, there may be episodes when they seem to recognise others, which in fact they will do, albeit probably only briefly.

Some patients may experience hallucinations and delusions at this time. A hallucination is an impression that something is present when it is not, so they may hear voices or see things that are not really there. A delusion is a false belief that cannot be reasoned out of – for example, believing that there is someone locked in a cupboard or that their grandfather is still alive.

If someone with dementia seems to be in distress at this stage, it may be because of a medical condition, such as a urinary or respiratory infection, or they could have a surgical problem. They may also be depressed. So it is important not to attribute every change to the dementia, as there may be another trigger that is causing distress. It is important that the problem is identified and they receive the appropriate care.

It is likely that the person will become increasingly frail as other organs start to be affected by the ongoing ageing process. They may have difficulty with balance, so that they need help to walk, including the use of a wheelchair. At the most extreme level of incapacity they may need bed care.

Incontinence is an increasing concern, since the nervous control to bowel and bladder may be compromised.

Nutrition and hydration are of paramount importance, since the person may show no interest themselves in eating and drinking. It is important that they are taking enough nutrients for their body and their brain. Similarly, it is vital that they take enough fluids, since dehydration can worsen the effects of dementia by altering the electrolyte levels of the body. That is, the sodium, potassium, calcium and chloride levels can all be affected by the state of hydration, which in turn can affect the way neurones operate to transmit their vital impulses sending information to and from the brain.

KEY POINTS

- The average length of life after diagnosis is 8–10 years.
- The older a person is at diagnosis, the shorter the length of time they may live. A 60-year-old may live 20–25 years, but a 90-year-old may only live two or three years more.
- The length of time one may live with dementia seems to correlate to the time of diagnosis. The earlier the diagnosis is made, the sooner any potential treatment can be started and the sooner care can be put in place to keep the person in good health.
- The reason that people with dementia die is that in the late stage they become unable to cope by themselves and become bedbound and dependent on others, eventually losing the ability to swallow. This leads to a risk of aspiration

pneumonia, from inhaling food or vomit into the lungs. Their declining health and other coexistent conditions may predispose them to infections.

The different types of dementia

As mentioned earlier, dementia is not one condition, but is an umbrella term used for a group of brain disorders that cause a deterioration of intellectual faculties, such as memory, concentration and judgement. We shall look at them in more detail in the following chapters, but it is important to differentiate between them, since they each have different pathologies, different features and may have different patterns of progression, and thus they may need different treatments.

Chapter 4

Alzheimer's disease

Alzheimer's is a brain disease that causes 62 per cent of cases of dementia. It causes changes in the brain and a reduction in neurotransmitters, which are involved in sending messages between nerve cells.

KEY POINTS

- Alzheimer's disease affects over 15 million people worldwide.
- Alzheimer's disease affects 465,000 people in the UK.
- The risk of developing Alzheimer's disease doubles every five years after the age of 65 years.
- In the UK, there are more than 16,000 people under the age of 65 years with Alzheimer's disease.
- It causes about a third of cases of early onset dementia (there are currently more than 40,000 people with early onset dementia in the UK).
- There is no known cure for Alzheimer's disease, but there are treatments that may slow down the onward progression of the condition.
- Alzheimer's disease is progressive.

- Alzheimer's disease was described by Alois Alzheimer in 1901, but he did not call it by that name. The name was first used by his colleague Emil Kraepelin in a textbook. Alzheimer had specifically described findings in the brain of a woman aged 51 years. Kraepelin wrote that there were two types of dementia, presenile and senile. He named the presenile variant after his colleague, and so for many decades Alzheimer's disease referred specifically to presenile dementia.

- Nowadays, Alzheimer's disease is considered to be a specific type of dementia that can occur at various ages, but which is commoner as age increases. Early onset Alzheimer's disease is generally regarded as the same condition occurring before the age of 65 years.

The 'disease of forgetfulness' – the first case described by Dr Alzheimer

In November 1901 Frau Auguste Deter, the 51-year-old wife of railway worker Karl Deter, was admitted to the City Hospital for the Mentally Ill and Epileptics in Frankfurt, Germany. Karl had been forced to give up work to look after his wife, whose behaviour had dramatically changed. She had developed extreme jealousy directed at her husband; she had problems with memory, reading and writing, and was prone to screaming at night.

Dr Alois Alzheimer, the medical director, examined her and made these case notes. His questions are recorded in italics, her answers are in inverted commas, and his observations are in parentheses.

(She sits on the bed with a helpless expression.)
What is your name?
'Auguste.'
What is your family name?
'Auguste.'
What is your husband's name?
'Ah, my husband.'
(She looks as if she didn't understand the question.)
Are you married?
'To Auguste.'
Mrs D?
'Yes, yes, Auguste D.'
How long have you been here?
(She seems to be trying to remember.)
'Three weeks.'
What is this?
(I show her a pencil.)
'A pen.'
(I show her a purse, key, diary and cigar, which are answered correctly.)

(At lunch she eats cauliflower and pork.)
What are you eating?
'Spinach.'
(When she was chewing meat and asked what she was doing, she answered potatoes and horseradish. When objects are shown to her, she does not remember after a short time which objects have been shown. In between she always speaks about twins. When she is asked to write, she holds the book in such a way that one has the impression that she has a loss in the right visual field. Asked to write Auguste D., she tries to write Mrs and forgets the rest. It is necessary to repeat every word.)

Her condition deteriorated over the next five years. Her memory completely disappeared. She lost all social skills, could not speak and started to have hallucinations, when she saw or heard things that were not there. Eventually, she became unable to care for herself at all and had to have continuous nursing.

She died in 1906, by which time Dr Alzheimer was working in Munich with Dr Emil Kraepelin. When he heard about her death he requested the case notes and her brain for examination. Later that year, he presented her case and the results of his examination of her brain to a meeting of the South-west German Society of Alienists ('Alienist' was the term for psychiatrist). He referred to it as 'the disease of forgetfulness'.

He described two abnormalities in the brain. Firstly, the brain was shrunken and had lost many of its convolutions; then, on microscopic examination of brain tissue, he also found neurofibrillary tangles and senile plaques.

KEY POINTS

The following are found in the brains of all Alzheimer's disease patients:

- Atrophy (shrinkage) of the brain
- Neurofibrillary tangles
- Amyloid plaques.
- Some of these changes are also found in the brains of people with other dementias.

Atrophy

Atrophy is the pathological term for shrinkage of an organ. Shrinkage of the brain is one of the main features of Alzheimer's disease. It seems to be most marked during the early stages of the disease in the temporal lobes of the brain, specifically the hippocampus (mentioned in Chapter 2, *Understand the brain*) which is associated with memory and information recall. Later it affects the whole of the brain; we refer to this as global atrophy.

Neurofibrillary tangles

The tangles that Alzheimer found on microscopic examination are the result of excessive tau protein causing cell death. The microtubules which form the axon of the individual neurones collapse and clump together to produce the tangled appearance. This seems to come about because of abnormal and excessive tau, the protein required by the nerve cells to maintain their shape, causing them to lose their normal function. The normal connections with other neighbouring cells are lost amid the tangle.

Senile plaques

Beta amyloid is another protein produced by nerve cells. It is formed when a much larger protein called amyloid precursor protein is broken down. The beta amyloid is laid down as clumps in the brains of Alzheimer's disease patients. These are known as amyloid plaques.

Fewer neurotransmitters

In Alzheimer's disease there is a depletion in the amount of the neurotransmitter acetylcholine. Whether this is a cause or an effect is not clear. Results of trying to boost acetylcholine in the brain have been disappointing.

The effect of all these changes is to disrupt the way that information is passed around the brain. Parts of the brain shrink as cells die and the function of those parts of the brain diminish, until eventually cognitive abilities disappear, emotions change and the personality seems to disappear.

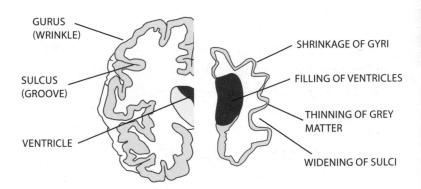

GURUS (WRINKLE)

SULCUS (GROOVE)

VENTRICLE

SHRINKAGE OF GYRI

FILLING OF VENTRICLES

THINNING OF GREY MATTER

WIDENING OF SULCI

Figure 7

KEY POINTS

In Alzheimer's disease there is:

- Global atrophy (shrinkage) of the brain
- Shrinkage of the gyri (the ridges or folds)
- Widening of the sulci (the crevices)
- Enlargement and filling up of the ventricles
- Thinning of the grey matter.

Two proteins are found in the brains of Alzheimer's patients:

- Beta amyloid produces plaques or clumps.
- Tau protein produces neurofibrillary tangles.

Some theories about the cause of Alzheimer's disease

Despite knowing something about the pathological changes that occur, we still do not have a clear picture of what causes Alzheimer's. There are several theories, each of which may play a part.

Genetic predisposition

People are understandably concerned about their own chance of developing Alzheimer's disease if a member of their family has the condition, or if a forebear died from it.

Several genes have been discovered to be associated with early onset Alzheimer's disease. One is involved in the function of the amyloid precursor protein (APP). It is found in chromosome 21, the same one associated with the commonest type of Down's syndrome. Two others found on chromosomes 1 and 14 are also involved in amyloid formation. They are called the presenilin genes, PS1 and PS2. PS1 is found on chromosome 14 and PS2 on chromosome 1. It has to be said, however, that these three genes are all quite rare and only account for about 10 per cent of cases of early onset Alzheimer's disease.

Population studies on Alzheimer's disease suggest that in late onset Alzheimer's disease 50–70 per cent of cases have an inherited tendency, although the genes involved have not been identified. This means that if Alzheimer's is in the family, the individual should modify their lifestyle to reduce other factors that could predispose them to the disease. We will look at this in Chapter 15 (*What can you do to reduce your risk of dementia?*).

Inflammation

In addition to the amyloid plaques, neurofibrillary tangles and brain atrophy mentioned above, the brains of Alzheimer's disease patients often show features of inflammation. This makes it possible that some viral illness could have triggered an inflammatory process in their brain.

In addition, scientists have discovered that the level of the COX-2 enzyme, known to be involved in the inflammation process, is found to be raised in certain parts of the brains of people with Alzheimer's disease. It is not conclusive as yet, but this may indicate that inflammation plays a part in the production of beta amyloid and the build-up of senile plaques in Alzheimer's disease. Aspirin is known to inhibit this enzyme and several clinical trials suggest that regular low-dose aspirin may reduce the risk of Alzheimer's disease by up to 23 per cent.[6]

Free radicals

In many metabolic processes where oxidation takes place, free radicals are produced. These are atoms or groups of atoms with an odd number of unpaired electrons. These very reactive radicals can start chain reactions, in the way that rows of dominoes tumble into one another, resulting in damage to cell components such as the DNA and the cell membranes. You can think of this as being rather like leaving a rubber band exposed to the air for a long time; it becomes friable and frayed. If you think of that happening to cell membranes, the insides of vessels and the tissues of the body, then you can see how the effects can be far-reaching.

There is much interest in antioxidants in food. These are natural chemicals that aid in the prevention of cell damage (the common pathway for inflammation), ageing and a whole host of degenerative diseases. They do this by mopping up free radicals. Much of the research suggests that diet can play a role in the prevention of heart disease, stroke and vascular dementia.

The tau hypothesis

It has been established that neurofibrillary tangles occur earlier than amyloid plaques, leading to what is known as the tau hypothesis. This suggests that the production of abnormal and excessive tau protein is the main process leading to the death of cells and the degenerative process that causes the other changes in Alzheimer's disease.

Aluminium and other metals

Over the years various metals have been suspected to play a role in the development of Alzheimer's disease. Aluminium was the first, when it was found that many people with Alzheimer's disease had trace amounts of aluminium in their brains at post-mortem examination. These findings have not been conclusively demonstrated since, equally, the brains of many other people with Alzheimer's contained no aluminium. The possibility is still under investigation, but the current thinking is that there is no need to avoid aluminium utensils or aluminium foil in cooking. An individual at increased risk, however, may feel it is worth reducing possible risk by avoiding drinks from aluminium cans or avoiding using aluminium foil, among other things.

Zinc is another metal that has been under investigation, without conclusive evidence one way or the other. Indeed, some results are downright confusing. For example, some studies have found that diets with low zinc may be associated with Alzheimer's, whereas others suggest that high levels may be damaging.

Copper has also come into question, since copper piping is used so commonly for plumbing. Again, no conclusive results have been found and the current thinking is that there is no reason for concern.

Most of the theories about metals revolve around the effect of trace amounts of metals causing interference with amyloid metabolism, leading to potential plaque formation in the brain. Clearly more research is needed.

The hygiene hypothesis

This is a relatively recent hypothesis, which suggests that our attention to hygiene and the desire to make our environment as germ-free as possible could in fact be predisposing people to Alzheimer's disease.

It has been observed that when children are brought up in households with pets they are less likely to develop allergies. In addition, various studies have shown that exposure to certain germs helps to prevent allergies, asthma and autoimmune disorders such as diabetes mellitus type 1 and inflammatory bowel disease. Lack of exposure can increase the risk of those conditions.

A study from Cambridge University looked at exposure to certain germs and the incidence of Alzheimer's disease in 192 countries.[7] They found that those countries with the lowest exposure to germs, because of high levels of sanitation, actually had higher rates of Alzheimer's disease.

Those countries with clean water supplies have a 9 per cent higher rate of Alzheimer's than countries where less than 50 per cent of the population have access to clean water. Also countries with the lowest levels of infectious diseases have 12 per cent higher rates of Alzheimer's than those with the highest levels of infectious diseases.

The postulate is that some exposure to bacteria is needed to stimulate the immune system, which in turn could tie in with the inflammation theory about Alzheimer's disease.

Glutamate excitotoxicity

Glutamate is the main excitatory neurotransmitter in the brain. It is involved in memory, thinking and learning. However, it has been found that too much glutamate overstimulates the cells. This happens because glutamate allows calcium to flow into the nerve cells, producing 'over-excitation', which has been found to lead to cell degeneration and cell death. This is called excitotoxic cell death and is thought to be one of the causes of various types of dementia, including Huntington's disease, Alzheimer's and vascular dementia.

The main features of Alzheimer's disease

The three stages of dementia outlined in the last chapter give a guide to how the condition progresses. The following symptoms are generally found in most cases of Alzheimer's disease. As we shall see in the following sections on other types of dementia, each type has its own dominant symptoms.

- Slow onset

- Often mild symptoms to begin with

- Steady and progressive memory loss

- Language and communication difficulties

- Decline in the ability to reason

- Decline in the ability to concentrate

- The loop phenomenon

- Poor judgement-making

- Indifference to self

- Progressive reduction in ability to care for themselves.

Four different presentations of Alzheimer's disease

In 2011 the National Institute on Aging and the Alzheimer's Association asked a working group to revise the criteria for Alzheimer's disease.[8] They concluded that there were four common but different presentations of Alzheimer's disease that could be seen. This is quite a useful way of looking at the condition, because there seem to be different ways in which it can present in its earliest stage.

Amnesic – the primary symptoms are impairment of memory plus another cognitive impairment.

Executive dysfunction – the primary symptoms are impairment of judgement and reasoning ability.

Posterior cortical atrophy (see below) – the primary difficulty is impairment of spatial cognition, which may express itself in trouble doing arithmetic or being able to do up shoelaces.

Language presentation – where the primary difficulty is in word finding and communication.

Gladys, my first case

I started my medical career intending to be a psychiatrist. I worked in a general psychiatric hospital, admitting and looking after patients with all types of mental illness. My very first patient was the 70-year-old widow of a bank manager. She was admitted to hospital for initial observation because she was finding it difficult to manage at home on her own. Her son, a solicitor, attended on her admission.

Gladys was well dressed, albeit with what seemed an eccentric combination of clothes. She was irritable and did not see why she had been brought to hospital. She felt that there was nothing wrong with her and that it was all her son's fault. What exactly was his fault she would not say.

Her son described her as having been temperamentally mercurial all of her life; that is, she was unpredictable and could go from being cheerful to very angry. He said that over the previous six months or so she had become more irritable, her memory had deteriorated, and she had been unable to manage her home. On occasions he had been called by her at different times of the night and had even been called by her neighbour because she had wandered out of her home at night in inappropriate clothing.

We used group therapy on the unit, which involved all of the patients. The aim was to explore how everyone was feeling and to involve everyone in the group. Over the next few months Gladys's ability to function in the group deteriorated. She could not concentrate, became less able to communicate and ultimately became totally confused by proceedings. Eventually, she was unable to look after herself and had to be accompanied by a nurse everywhere.

Finally, she became bed-bound, unable to recognise her son, the staff or any of the other patients. I moved to another job, but returned to the hospital to do outpatient clinics. I kept an interest in her case and was sad when she died a few months later.

A post-mortem examination confirmed the clinical diagnosis that she had Alzheimer's disease. This was a fairly rapid deterioration, but one that was typical of the deterioration of memory, intellect and personality which is found in Alzheimer's disease.

KEY POINTS

- On average a patient with Alzheimer's disease will live for 8–10 years with the condition.
- A person with Alzheimer's in their 60s and 70s can expect to live 7–10 years.
- A person with Alzheimer's in their 90s can expect to live about two or three years.

Posterior cortical atrophy

This is a relatively rare variant of Alzheimer's disease, which is also sometimes called Benson's syndrome after Dr Frank Benson, who first described it in 1988.[9] It mainly affects the posterior part of the brain, rather than showing the global atrophy of typical Alzheimer's disease.

Sir Terry Pratchett, the bestselling author, was diagnosed with this condition in 2007. He is still able to write, because it does not affect those cognitive functions involved in imagination, communication and writing. However, it does have a progressive course, affecting vision, spelling and arithmetic.

There is also considerable variation in symptoms within PCA, which leads some specialists to consider that it is in fact a separate condition from Alzheimer's disease.

Hippocampal-sparing Alzheimer's disease

This is another variant that is thought to account for up to 10 per cent of cases of Alzheimer's disease. In this situation the hippocampus is spared, so memory loss is not a feature. Instead, they often have personality changes or behavioural problems and sometimes movement problems. It tends to occur at a younger age than typical Alzheimer's disease and is commoner in males than females. Its course tends to be faster and death occurs sooner than in typical Alzheimer's disease.

This variant is in need of further research, since many people with this condition may be undiagnosed or else diagnosed with another condition. It is thought that some of the drugs used for Alzheimer's disease could work well for these patients.

Chapter 5

Vascular dementia

This is the second most common type of dementia, accounting for about 17–20 per cent of cases. Vascular dementia is caused when strokes occur, or when the small blood vessels that supply the brain fur up and become blocked.

> **KEY POINT**
>
> More than 110,000 people in the UK are affected by vascular dementia, of which there are several different types.

The blood supply of the brain

The brain needs a continuous supply of blood. As mentioned in the first chapter, the blood supply to the brain was discovered by Dr Thomas Willis in the mid-seventeenth century. Essentially, the two internal carotid arteries in the front of the neck pass up into the skull and form a ring with vessels from the basilar artery, which is itself formed from two vertebral arteries which pass up the back of the neck into the back of the skull. This ring, called the Circle of Willis, is located underneath the brain. Smaller arteries then branch off from it and travel upwards to supply specific parts of the brain.

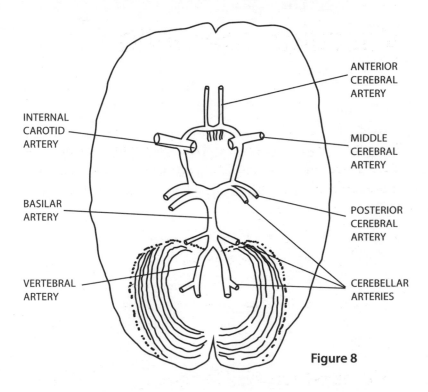

ANTERIOR CEREBRAL ARTERY

INTERNAL CAROTID ARTERY

MIDDLE CEREBRAL ARTERY

BASILAR ARTERY

POSTERIOR CEREBRAL ARTERY

VERTEBRAL ARTERY

CEREBELLAR ARTERIES

Figure 8

Stroke

A stroke is the name given to a brain attack in which an area of the brain is deprived of its blood supply. The blood supplies the brain with oxygen and nutrients, including glucose. If the blood supply is cut off to a part of the brain then the delicate brain cells will start to become damaged and quickly die off. This takes place within a mere six minutes, so time is of the essence.

It is important to appreciate that **a stroke is always a serious event and should be treated as a medical emergency**. Permanent damage to the brain can occur, or even death.

The blood supply is affected in two main ways:

Ischaemia

This means that a blockage occurs in a blood vessel. Generally this is the result of cholesterol plaques building up inside the vessel, caused essentially by a hardening of the arteries.

There are two ways an ischaemic stroke can occur:

- If a plaque on a brain blood vessel ruptures then a clot rapidly forms around the damaged area. If this is large enough to block the flow of blood then the part of the brain supplied by that blood vessel may be damaged.

- If a clot forms in another part of the body and flows along the blood's circulation to lodge in a narrowed part of an artery supplying the brain, this clot is called an embolus and also produces ischaemia.

Haemorrhage

This is when a bleed into the brain itself occurs when a blood vessel bursts.

When someone has a stroke it may be possible on the basis of the clinical examination to deduce which part of the brain has been affected. Further investigation, including various types of scan, may pinpoint the site of the lesion and determine the nature of the damage.

These are the arteries and the areas of the brain they supply:

- Anterior cerebral arteries – supply the front of the brain and the motor and sensory areas for the lower part of the body. A blocked anterior cerebral artery may cause paralysis and sensory deficit on the opposite side of the body from the hips down. There can also be incontinence of the bowel or the bladder. Since these arteries also supply the frontal area some personality change can occur.

- Middle cerebral arteries – supply a large part of the brain including the corpus striatum, which is involved in regulating our movements, and thus can result in a wide variety of problems. These affect the areas involved in speech, swallowing and language function. A stroke affecting the middle cerebral artery can also cause a specific visual defect called hemianopsia, in which the loss of half of the visual field in each eye is the result. For example, if someone has a stroke affecting their right middle cerebral artery they will experience loss of their left field of view in both eyes.

- Posterior cerebral arteries – supply a lot of the hind part of the brain. Since this area has a large part to play in vision, there can be a wide variety of visual problems associated with haemorrhage in these arteries.

- Cerebellar arteries – supply the cerebellum, so they are often associated with ataxia, or balance and coordination problems.

Mini-stroke or transient cerebral ischaemic attack, TIA

Mini-strokes or transient ischaemic attacks must not be regarded as insignificant. These are ischaemic brain attacks which are reversible and clear up within 24 hours. But they are just as important to recognise, investigate and treat as are full-blown strokes.

They can produce the same signs and symptoms as a full stroke or they may produce very minimal signs, such as a slight drooping of the eyelid or the mouth. They must never be ignored. People may be tempted to just wait and see if the symptoms disappear, but one can never be sure without a physical examination by a doctor and, if needed, investigation as to whether it is a TIA or a developing stroke that is getting worse. Precious time may be wasted by delaying, so if the FAST test described in the accompanying box is positive, then it is time to call for urgent help.

Even if there has been a cluster of symptoms that have subsequently reversed themselves, these should still be checked out by your doctor. Although a TIA has been reversed, it could be followed by a much more severe and even life-threatening stroke. Moreover, repeated TIAs can result in vascular dementia, so they need to be investigated and prevented.

THE FAST TEST

The Stroke Association recommends the FAST test, which alerts you to the things to look for and the action you must take if someone appears to have suffered a stroke. FAST stands for:

FACIAL weakness – ask the person to smile, and look to see if the mouth is drooping on one side.

ARM weakness – can the person raise both arms?

SPEECH problems – can the person speak clearly, without slurring? Do they understand what you are saying?

TIME TO CALL – the emergency number (999 in the UK)

Quite simply, if the person fails any of these tests there is enough evidence to suspect that they are having a stroke. The faster that you get help, the better the prospect of minimising any damage to their brain. This will improve their chances of recovery. It may even save their life.

KEY POINTS

Strokes vary immensely:

- Ischaemic strokes can be fast or slow to develop. Symptoms may progress gradually as the ischaemic area undergoes swelling and inflammation, so that the extent of the stroke is not immediately apparent. This is often called a stroke in evolution, since the stroke is continuing to evolve.
- Haemorrhagic strokes are sudden. They are more likely to be associated with a headache, as they are caused by a burst blood vessel. And they are more likely to be catastrophic than ischaemic strokes.
- Mini-strokes, correctly known as transient ischaemic attacks or TIAs, can occur without the individual knowing. These can lead to one of the types of vascular dementia.

The different types of vascular dementia

Just as there are different ways that the brain can be affected by stroke, so too there are different types of vascular dementia.

Single infarct dementia

This occurs when there is a large stroke. Damage occurs to the brain and the cells in that area die off. The name for the death of tissue is infarction.

Multi-infarct dementia

This occurs when damage to the brain occurs from a succession of small strokes or mini-strokes. The person may not be aware that they have occurred, so that no physical effects are experienced, such as paralysis. Each subsequent small infarction of part of the brain adds to the effects of previous ones, so that the brain becomes affected in various places.

Subcortical vascular dementia

This sort of dementia occurs when there is damage to many small blood vessels deep inside the brain. This tends to occur in longstanding conditions, such as atherosclerosis (hardening of the arteries) in old age, diabetes and hypertension, which have caused narrowing of the blood vessels. When a clot forms in one of these small, deep vessels it will cause a lacunar stroke.

The term is used because the brain typically shows a lacuna, which is Latin for 'empty space'. This space can take years to form after the original stroke. It occurs because when one of these little blood vessels is blocked, it is like blocking a cul-de-sac, so that the small area beyond the block eventually just melts away to become a space, like the hole in a sponge.

Lacunar strokes account for about 25 per cent of ischaemic strokes, which means that they account for roughly 20 per cent of all strokes. They may even occur 'silently' in that a person may not be aware of having had a stroke. When there are many of these lacunar strokes, the brain can become like a sponge with lacunae throughout, and this can lead to subcortical dementia. That is, the damage is occurring below the cortex, deep in the brain substance, inside the white matter of the brain. This will affect the wiring of the brain to the body and will produce a lot of physical symptoms before it eventually leads to a loss of mental function.

This condition usually presents between the ages of 54 and 66 years of age. It is sometimes called Binswanger's disease, having been first described in 1902 by Dr Otto Binswanger, a Swiss psychiatrist and neurologist.

Mixed dementia

This is a combination of both Alzheimer's disease and vascular dementia. Such patients will experience and manifest features of both types of dementia, so that there will be both physical symptoms and deterioration of mental function. Memory problems may not be so marked as in typical Alzheimer's disease, depending upon which areas of the brain have been affected.

This condition accounts for about 10 per cent of all dementias.

Risk factors for vascular dementia

The main risk factor for the development of vascular dementia is stroke. Therefore, all of the factors that put people at risk of having a heart attack or a stroke, also put them at risk of vascular dementia.

- Hypertension – this is the name for high blood pressure

- Raised cholesterol

- Irregular heart function, especially atrial fibrillation

- Smoking

- Excess alcohol

- Diabetes mellitus

- Lack of exercise

- Obesity

- Head injury history – either a single or multiple, as can occur in contact sports.

Additionally:

- Race can increase the risk. Vascular dementia is commoner in Asian and Black Caribbean people, who are also at greater risk of developing hypertension and diabetes.

- Genetic predisposition: some people are at greater risk as a result of their genetic make-up. One such condition is a rare inherited genetic disorder called 'Cerebral autosomal dominant arteriopathy with subcortical infarcts and leukoencephalopathy', usually referred to as CADASIL. It is associated with frequent migraines and repeated strokes and starts at a young age, about thirty. It can be diagnosed by blood and tissue sampling. There is no specific treatment, but antiplatelet drugs like aspirin, clopidogrel and dipyridamole may be used to reduce risk of having a stroke.

The main features of vascular dementia

It is not always easy to differentiate between the dementias. Whereas Alzheimer's disease is characterised by memory problems (Alzheimer himself described it as the disease of forgetfulness), patients with vascular dementia may or may not have memory disturbance. Their symptoms entirely depend upon which parts of the brain are affected.

It is highly likely that those with vascular dementia will have physical symptoms, too, since the parts of the brain that are responsible for moving the body – the motor parts – are likely to be affected.

Thus, vascular dementia symptoms may include:

- Emotional changes

- Communication and language difficulties

- Weakness or paralysis of one side of the body

- Incontinence of bladder or bowel

- Disturbance of balance.

The progression of vascular dementia is different from Alzheimer's disease. There is usually a sudden onset, relating to a stroke. This demonstrates that there is underlying cerebrovascular disease. Then there is often a definite deterioration associated with each stroke. Thus, there can be a stepwise course, in that the progression of the disease is not gradual and continuous, as is Alzheimer's, but occurs over a series of discrete, sudden changes, each one associated with a stroke or TIA. The development of physical symptoms, like paralysis or weakness of one side of the body, as occurs with strokes, will be more marked than with typical Alzheimer's disease.

This situation may be seen in patients with repeated mini-strokes or TIAs. They will deteriorate then seem to experience some recovery until the next episode. There will then be the same three-stage deterioration outlined in Chapter 3.

KEY POINTS

- Vascular dementia is a manifestation of cerebrovascular disease.
- It is slightly commoner in men than women.
- There tends to be a stepwise progression of the condition, with deterioration occurring in discrete, sudden changes rather than gradually, and with each step or change relating to a stroke or definite brain event.
- This kind of dementia is related to cerebrovascular disease, so treatment of the cerebrovascular disease can prevent further cerebral infarcts and potentially further deterioration.

Albert – a case of vascular dementia

This case comes from my early days in general practice. Albert was a 66-year-old man who started having falling attacks, when for no obvious reason he would feel dizzy and overbalance. Shortly after they started, he noticed that he could feel confused and his wife told him that he kept asking the same questions over and over.

Then he had a definite mini-stroke from which he made a good recovery. Again, the loop phenomenon occurred and he would repeat the same question to his wife. He was hypertensive and was treated for this and given aspirin to try to reduce the risk of further TIAs.

His mental state started to deteriorate rapidly. His memory function deteriorated, he couldn't concentrate and he stopped doing his gardening, an activity he had loved.

There then followed three strokes in fairly rapid succession, after each of which his mental processes further deteriorated. Within two years he needed continuous nursing for his vascular dementia.

The treatment of vascular dementia

In treatment, the emphasis is on preventing further cerebral infarcts which would worsen the dementia. This may mean the use of agents like aspirin. We shall look at drug treatments in Chapter 12 (*Medical treatment*). Cognitive enhancers are not currently licensed for treating vascular dementia.

Very importantly, treatment will involve help with rehabilitation after stroke, and such measures as can maintain the well-being and independence of the individual as much as possible. This may involve physiotherapy, occupational therapy, and speech and language therapy.

Psychological help may be available if there are behavioural problems or if the person's ability to perform day-to-day tasks is affected. Psychological support and cognitive behavioural therapy may help.

Group therapy with arts and crafts, music and reminiscence therapy can also help. Essentially, reminiscence therapy uses photographs and things from the person's past to rekindle memory and help with emotions.

Chapter 6

Dementia with Lewy bodies and Parkinson's disease dementia

In this chapter we are going to look at two of the less common but very important types of dementia. They are different from both Alzheimer's disease and vascular dementia, although they do have some features in common with Alzheimer's. These conditions are dementia with Lewy bodies (DLB) and Parkinson's disease dementia (PDD). But there is some overlap between these two, so along with Parkinson's disease itself (without dementia) they are often referred to as the spectrum of Lewy body disorders.

Dementia with Lewy bodies, DLB

This form of dementia is less common than both Alzheimer's disease and vascular dementia, but it still affects a significant number of people. It is sometimes referred to as Lewy body dementia (LBD). The two terms mean the same condition.

- Dementia with Lewy bodies accounts for 4 per cent of all dementias (although some estimates put the figure at 10 per cent, because it is often misdiagnosed).

- Its incidence rises with age, so that according to the Lewy Body Society it affects 5 per cent of all people by the age of 85 years.

- In the UK there are approximately 100,000 people suffering from dementia with Lewy bodies, also known as Lewy body dementia.

- It has symptoms in common with Alzheimer's disease and Parkinson's disease. Parkinson's disease is a progressive neurological condition that affects movement.

Parkinson's disease dementia, PDD

This is a rarer form of dementia, accounting for about 2 per cent of all new cases of dementia. To put it into perspective, first we have to consider Parkinson's disease. This is a progressive neurological disorder that affects movement, which is caused by insufficient dopamine in parts of the brain called the basal ganglia. Dopamine is a neurotransmitter.

The condition tends to produce slowness of movement and a coarse tremor most marked at rest, which manifests as the classic 'pill-rolling' tremor, as if the person is rolling a pill between their fingers. It also can produce a mask-like or expressionless face, and a reduced ability to blink.

It was first described by Dr James Parkinson in his medical paper 'An essay on the Shaking Palsy', now considered one of the classics of medical literature.

- Parkinson's disease affects one person in 500.

- There are about 127,000 people with Parkinson's disease in the UK.

- The onset is usually at the age of 50 years or over.

- People with Parkinson's disease have about a 25 per cent risk of developing Parkinson's disease dementia.

Parkinson's disease dementia, PDD, is diagnosed when someone who has had Parkinson's disease for some time starts to develop symptoms of dementia.

KEY POINTS

- Dementia with Lewy bodies, DLB, is diagnosed when someone with dementia develops symptoms of Parkinson's disease which affect their movements, or when someone develops symptoms of dementia and Parkinson's disease at the same time.

- Parkinson's disease dementia, PDD, is diagnosed when someone who has had Parkinson's disease for some time starts to develop symptoms of dementia.

- The diagnosis is usually made by a specialist.

Lewy bodies and the Lewy body spectrum

Lewy bodies are tiny deposits of protein found in nerve cells. Some of them have what appears to be a halo around them. They were first discovered by Dr Friedrich (later Frederic) Lewy (1885–1950), a Jewish German-born American neurologist, when he was studying the brains of people who had suffered from Parkinson's disease.

They have since been found in the brains of patients with Parkinson's disease and Parkinson's disease dementia, and are very characteristic of dementia with Lewy bodies. Their presence is not diagnostic of Parkinson's disease dementia or of dementia with Lewy bodies, since they can also be found in other types of dementia; but they are usually associated with lowered levels of the neurotransmitters acetylcholine and dopamine.

Gradually, in a person with PDD brain cells die off and the shrinkage of the brain occurs that is common to all dementias. But the symptoms experienced by the individual depend upon where the Lewy bodies are found in the brain. Thus:

- Lewy bodies in the base of the brain – will tend to produce Parkinson's disease, which has the following features:
    - movement disorders
    - shaking
    - slowness of movement.

- Lewy bodies in the cerebral cortex – will tend to produce dementia with Lewy bodies, with the following features:
    - memory problems
    - cognitive problems
    - hallucinations.

Symptoms in dementia with Lewy bodies

The start of the condition, like that of Alzheimer's, may be very subtle. It may simply involve memory problems or episodes of confusion. It cannot be overemphasised, however, that the earliest possible diagnosis is needed to control symptoms. The correct diagnosis is important, since medication can be troublesome, as we shall soon consider.

Dementia

The presence of dementia is the usual starting point. The person may seem to have the typical memory problems and lack of concentration of Alzheimer's disease.

Parkinson's symptoms

This can start with a tremor, then shaking during movements of the hand. In some people there may be the classic 'pill-rolling' movement of the hand, as if one is rolling a small pill between finger and thumb. The face may become relatively expressionless. There may be a stiffness or rigidity of muscles, and movements may seem jerky or cogwheel-like. There may be a shuffling of the feet, general slowness of movement and a tendency to fall due to poor balance.

Hallucinations and delusions

These are quite characteristic of dementia with Lewy bodies, but are less common with Alzheimer's disease and vascular dementia. A hallucination is an impression that something is present when in reality it is not. Thus, a visual hallucination means that someone sees something that is not really there. For example, seeing someone sitting opposite when there is no one present. An auditory hallucination is when one hears voices or other noises that are not there.

A delusion is a false belief in something that cannot be reasoned away. These often follow hallucinations. For example, if someone has the visual hallucination that there is someone who regularly comes and sits opposite them, or who comes and switches on their television set, then they may come to believe that other people are living with them when in reality they live on their own.

Disturbed sleep

This, too, is characteristic of dementia with Lewy bodies. The person often sleeps in the daytime without any problem, but night sleep is disturbed. They may experience nightmares, cry out, get up and hallucinate. Their eyes may move rapidly under their eyelids. This symptom is called *rapid eye movement sleep behaviour disorder*. It can be highly distressing for the bed partner of someone with DLB.

Sensitivity to drugs

This is an important point since some drugs that are given to deal with the distressing hallucinations and delusions and behavioural problems associated with the dementia may make Parkinson's symptoms worse. Conversely, some drugs that are given to deal with Parkinson's may worsen a psychosis; that is, they may worsen the hallucinations and delusions while also causing other symptoms to arise. This is why treatment should be initiated by a specialist.

Dementia with Lewy bodies and Parkinson's disease dementia – the differences

The difference between the two conditions may be subtle and there is still debate as to whether they are indeed separate conditions. At this time there are not thought to be any major differences in pathology. It may be simply that different parts of the brain are affected by a similar process involving the production of Lewy bodies.

Differentiation between them is usually done by a specialist in elderly psychiatry or a psychogeriatrician. At the moment the distinction between the conditions is based upon the clinical history and the first appearance of the various symptoms. Thus:

- Parkinson's disease dementia is diagnosed if dementia develops in someone who has had Parkinson's disease for longer than 12 months.

- Dementia with Lewy bodies is diagnosed if dementia develops before or at the same time as Parkinson's disease.

- There is a 12-month diagnostic rule that says if the dementia occurs within 12 months of the start of the Parkinsonism, it is diagnosed as dementia with Lewy bodies.

KEY POINTS

- Early diagnosis of dementia with Lewy bodies by a specialist is important.
- Hallucinations and delusions are characteristic features of dementia with Lewy bodies.
- Rapid eye movement sleep behaviour disorder is characteristic of dementia with Lewy bodies.
- With adequate treatment one can live well with dementia with Lewy bodies.
- Dementia with Lewy bodies is a progressive disease that shortens the lifespan. The average age of survival is 5–8 years from diagnosis.

General treatment in dementia with Lewy bodies

Speech therapy may be helpful for low voice volume and poor enunciation. Speech therapy may also improve muscular strength and swallowing difficulties.

Occupational therapy may help maintain skills and promote function and independence. In addition, music and art therapy can reduce anxiety and improve mood.

Individual and family psychotherapy can be useful for learning strategies to manage emotional and behavioural symptoms and to help make plans that address individual and family concerns about the future.

Support groups may be helpful for caregivers and persons with LBD.

Medical treatment of dementia with Lewy bodies

The drug treatment of this type of dementia has to be started by a specialist. People with dementia with Lewy bodies may be very sensitive to some of the drugs that are used to treat both Alzheimer's disease and Parkinson's disease. They may also be sensitive to drugs bought over the counter, so it is always important to check with the GP before giving any type of drug.

Cognitive symptoms

The acetylcholinesterase inhibitors or ACEI drugs (see Chapter 12, *Medical treatment*) are used in mild and moderate stages of Alzheimer's disease, and may also be of great benefit in slowing the cognitive function deterioration in dementia with Lewy bodies. It is suggested by NICE, the National Institute for Health and Care Excellence, that acetylcholinesterase inhibitor drugs such as rivastigmine can reduce the cognitive decline in dementia with Lewy bodies.

Hallucinations

The antipsychotic or neuroleptic drugs (see Chapter 12, *Medical treatment*) may be used to control hallucinations and behavioural problems in Alzheimer's disease. However, they should be avoided in persons with LBD, because these patients often have 'neuroleptic sensitivity', meaning that they overreact to these drugs.

It has been found that the acetylcholinesterase inhibitor drugs can control hallucinations in dementia with Lewy bodies.

Movement symptoms

The movement symptoms of LBD may be improved by giving L-DOPA or levodopa, the drug used to treat Parkinson's disease. However, it is possible that this could worsen the hallucinations and delusions that are common in LBD. Therefore, if the movement problems are mild and not bothering the person too much, they are probably best left untreated.

Treatment of Parkinson's disease dementia

There are currently no treatments that slow down the damage caused by Parkinson's disease dementia. The focus is on alleviating any symptoms.

As with dementia with Lewy bodies, someone with Parkinson's disease dementia may be helped by speech therapy, occupational therapy, individual and family therapy and by attending support groups.

Cognitive symptoms

The acetylcholinesterase inhibitors or ACEI drugs which are used in mild and moderate stages of Alzheimer's disease may also be a great benefit in slowing the cognitive function deterioration in Parkinson's disease dementia.

Hallucinations

These are not as common in Parkinson's disease dementia as they are with dementia with Lewy bodies, yet they can occur. Antipsychotic or neuroleptic drugs (see Chapter 12, *Medical treatment*) may be used to control hallucinations and behavioural problems in Alzheimer's disease, but have to be used with great caution in people with Parkinson's disease dementia. They can cause worsening of the Parkinson's disease movement symptoms.

Movement symptoms

The movement symptoms can be improved by taking L-DOPA, but this can produce hallucinations.

REM sleep disorders

These may be helped by clonazepam, a benzodiazepine drug with anxiolytic (reduces anxiety), muscle-relaxant and sedative effects.

Chapter 7

Fronto-temporal dementia and other dementias

The types of dementia that we are going to cover in this chapter are rarer than those we have looked at before, but it is important to address them because their different causes and different patterns may produce different needs.

Fronto-temporal dementia, FTD

This is also sometimes known as Pick's disease, after its discoverer, Dr Arnold Pick. A professor of psychiatry at Prague, in 1892 he described a condition in which there is atrophy of the frontal and temporal lobes of the brain, resulting in dementia. The condition causes 2 per cent of all new cases of dementia in the UK.

The two areas of the brain that are mainly affected by this condition have major functions in shaping our personalities, so behavioural disorders and personality changes may be seen in this dementia.

This condition can be difficult to diagnose, because it often occurs at an earlier age than other dementias. Whereas most dementias occur after the age of 65 years, fronto-temporal dementia tends to start between the ages of 45 and 65 years. It is therefore a common cause of early onset dementia.

It can start considerably earlier, with cases having occurred in people in their twenties, and it can also occur in elderly people in their seventies and eighties.

The types of problems caused

It may help to recap on the functions of the frontal and temporal lobes.

- The frontal lobes (there is a right and a left frontal lobe) are where reasoning, calculation, problem solving and judgement take place. Thus they are command areas of the brain for behaviour. Broca's area, which controls speech, is usually in the frontal lobe.

- The temporal lobes are mainly concerned with memory, although also associated with emotions and speech. Wernicke's area, which controls language recognition, is located in the left hemisphere. Sound is also perceived in the temporal lobes.

- When these important parts of the brain suffer from nerve cell damage and loss of cells, the lobes shrink. The functions associated with them therefore deteriorate.

There are actually three variants of fronto-temporal dementia that can be seen:

Behaviour variant FTD

This is predominantly loss of frontal brain cells. It causes personality changes, lack of insight and lack of awareness of the consequences of actions. The individual makes poor judgements and may put him or herself in danger by failing to perceive risk. They can become uninhibited and neglectful of their self and personal hygiene.

Progressive nonfluent aphasia, PNFA

Here the dominant symptoms are difficulties with language, because both Broca's and Wernicke's areas are affected. The speech fluency is particularly affected. The person may make grammatical errors and hesitate between words. Aphasia means difficulty with speech, or non-speech.

Semantic dementia

This affects the temporal area associated with writing and the understanding of language, so that these skills are lost early in the process. This may precede memory disturbance.

The causes of fronto-temporal dementia

About 50 per cent of fronto-temporal dementia seems to be associated with tau protein pathology. The build-up of tau proteins in nerve cells can be seen on microscopic examination after post-mortem examination of the brain. Silver-staining is used to make them stand out as spherical clumps known as 'Pick bodies'.

Tau protein build-up can also be associated with other progressive neurological conditions, such as progressive supranuclear palsy (see below) and motor neurone disease.

In about 30–50 per cent of cases there is a family history of fronto-temporal dementia in a first-degree relative. Thus, a genetic cause seems to be at work in these cases.

Other, rarer types of dementia

Alcohol-related dementia

Alcohol generally has a complex effect on health. Small quantities seem to be beneficial, yet larger amounts predispose an individual to many conditions, including heart disease, stroke, liver disease and dementia.

Heavy drinkers often neglect their diet, the result being that they can develop thiamine deficiency. Thiamine is one of the B group vitamins, and prolonged deficiency seems to lead to damage to parts of the brainstem, which may result in two separate but related conditions (see below).

Wernicke's encephalopathy

This is an acute confusional state due to prolonged heavy drinking. It comes on suddenly and is associated with the four following features:

- Evidence of malnutrition – the person is underweight and looks undernourished.

- Involuntary, jerky eye movements – this is called nystagmus; the eyes move from side to side continuously.

- Impaired balance – this suggests disturbance of the cerebellum, the large structure at the back and the bottom of the brain, which controls movement and balance.

- Confusion.

This conditon is a medical emergency, necessitating hospital treatment and intravenous infusion of thiamine via a drip. It is possible to reverse the effects and prevent further brain damage, provided alcohol is stopped and the thiamine intake is maintained, but further heavy drinking may lead to further damage and possible dementia.

Korsakoff's syndrome

This syndrome was first described by the Russian psychiatrist Sergei Korsakoff (1854–1900) when he was studying the effects of alcoholism. It used to be referred to as Korsakoff's psychosis, because it produced profound short-term memory problems, as well as paranoia and in some patients a noticeable detachment from reality.

It is caused by damage to the mammillary bodies, which are small round areas on the undersurface of the brain. They are part of the limbic system (see Chapter 2, *Understand the brain*) and are important for gathering memories.

People with Korsakoff's syndrome exhibit the following:

- Confabulation – they lie to fill in gaps in their memory.

- Inability to learn new skills or to retain information.

- Lack of insight into their condition.

- Personality change – this can be any change in personality.

It is possible to reverse the changes brought about by this condition, so it is not the same process as Alzheimer's disease, where there is progressive deterioration. The treatment entails stopping drinking, improving diet and maintaining adequate thiamine intake. Unfortunately, many people with Korsakoff syndrome are homeless and may have drifted into a life habit of alcohol abuse.

KEY POINTS

The Royal College of Physicians recommends that:

- Men should not drink more than 21 units of alcohol a week.
- A unit is either a small measure of spirit, a small glass of wine or a half pint of beer or lager.
- Sensible drinking – the daily alcohol intake should not exceed 3–4 units for men.
- Women should not drink more than 14 units a week.
- Sensible drinking – the daily alcohol intake should not exceed 2–3 units for women.
- Continued drinking at the upper limit is not advised, and at least two alcohol-free days a week should be taken.
- As a rule of thumb, heavy drinking is defined as six units in six hours.

Normal pressure hydrocephalus

This is a condition in which the ventricles of the brain dilate and are filled up with cerebrospinal fluid. Hydrocephalus, which means 'water on the brain', is usually associated with a rise in pressure as measured by lumbar puncture. This excess fluid and increased pressure squeeze and damage the brain. It is a condition most often seen in infants and children, where the skull bones have not fused and the head therefore enlarges.

In normal pressure hydrocephalus, which can occur in adults, there is no such sustained pressure increase, although it is thought that in the early stages the pressure does rise. The problem comes about because the ventricles swell and put pressure on the brain.

Since the skull bones are fused in adulthood there is no way that the brain can expand, so damage will result. It produces:

- Dementia

- Unsteady gait

- Incontinence.

In 50 per cent of cases there is a known cause:

- Past head injury

- Past subarachnoid haemorrhage

- Cerebral tumour

- Past meningitis.

A neurosurgical operation involving the insertion of a shunt might reverse the condition. A shunt is a narrow tube inserted into the ventricle and threaded under the skin down through the neck. This drains excess cerebrospinal fluid (CSF) into another part of the body, such as the heart or abdomen.

Progressive supranuclear palsy, PSP

This is a rare condition in which the parts of the brain that control balance and movement are damaged. The person loses coordination and may develop a tendency to fall over. Speech is affected as are eye movements and sometimes swallowing. The cause is unknown.

It tends to affect people over the age of 60 years. As yet there is no cure, but some drugs may help to control symptoms.

The personality may change and once the condition is advanced, dementia may occur. However, memory may not be as badly affected as with other dementias and some insight may be retained.

Creutzfeldt-Jakob disease

This is a rare and ultimately fatal disease affecting the brain. It affects about 50 people in the UK every year. It is rapidly progressive, with death occurring usually within a year of the onset. It produces the following symptoms:

- Personality change

- Memory problems

- Balance difficulty

- Slurred speech

- Visual problems, possibly leading to blindness

- Ataxia – jerking movements and a staggering walk

- Progressive physical decline

- Progressive mental decline to dementia.

The disease is caused by a prion, an abnormal protein smaller than a virus, so there is some debate as to whether it can be called a life form. There are four subtypes of the disease, three of which usually occur after the age of 60. The fourth, variant CJD, which is caused by consuming infected meat, can affect young adults. It has similar features to bovine spongiform encephalopathy, or so called 'mad cow disease'.

There is no cure at this time and treatment involves symptomatic relief.

HIV-related dementia

About 10 per cent of people infected with the human immunodeficiency virus, which produces acquired immune deficiency syndrome, or AIDS, develop progressive mental decline leading to dementia.

Treatment of the condition with anti-retroviral drugs has considerably reduced the incidence of this outcome.

Huntington's disease

This is an inherited disease that profoundly affects the brain, causing progressive loss of mental functions, movement disorders and ultimately dementia. It was first described by George Huntington in 1872, after he had observed and examined the combined medical history of several generations of a family who manifested similar symptoms of movement disorder and progressive mental decline.

In Huntington's disease the cerebral cortex is affected to produce the mental decline but also to cause symptoms akin to schizophrenia. Depression and anxiety are also common with this condition. Moreover, patients begin to show poor judgement and often undergo a personality change. Their behaviour may start to seem bizarre and they may also become uninhibited.

The basal ganglia are also affected, the areas of the brain that control smooth movement and the same areas affected in Parkinson's disease. In Huntington's, the movement disorder is such that all manner of involuntary movements occur in all four limbs, as well as facial grimacing and movements of the trunk. The original name for the condition was Huntington's chorea, since chorea is the Greek word for dance.

The disease starts in early adulthood and progresses over 20 years or so. The person will ultimately require total nursing care.

It is caused by an inherited faulty gene. A parent with the gene will pass it on to half of their offspring. Anyone who has the faulty gene will develop the condition; this is referred to as an autosomal dominant pattern of inheritance. There is nothing that can be done to prevent the condition, but treatment can help alleviate some of its complications, such as depression and anxiety.

Corticobasal degeneration, CBD

This is a rare disease affecting the cortex and the basal ganglia. It is not known what causes it, but in common with other dementias it seems to relate to the build-up of unusual amounts of tau protein in the brain.

The condition starts with a movement disorder, taking the form of stiffness and jerkiness spreading from first one limb to all of the limbs at the same time as mental decline also sets in. There may be balance problems, as well as difficulty in speaking and swallowing.

There is no cure, but treatment with drugs may help alleviate symptoms. Physiotherapy, occupational therapy and speech therapy may also be helpful.

The condition is progressive, leading to death on average eight or nine years after onset.

Multiple sclerosis

This is a demyelinating condition, meaning that the sheath around nerve cells is lost. As a result the nerves do not transmit information and thus paralysis occurs of various parts of the body supplied by those nerves. There are two types of multiple sclerosis:

- Primary progressive

- Relapsing and remitting.

In some people with the condition, depending upon which parts of the nervous system are affected, there can be mental decline. It is unusual, however, for this to progress to the stage of dementia, though it may happen in a small number of cases.

Niemann-Pick disease type C

This is a rare inherited disorder which affects school-age children, in particular, but can also affect adults, too. The condition prevents the body from handling its cholesterol, which ultimately affects the nervous system, causing difficulty with movement and with swallowing. If onset is in adolescence or adulthood, it can lead to dementia. This can cause memory problems and difficulty concentrating. There is no effective treatment, although research is ongoing.

Chapter 8

Depression, delirium and mild cognitive impairment – things that can be confused with dementia

Now that we have looked at the different types of dementia, it is useful to look at reversible conditions that can be mistaken for dementia. Please note that word, 'reversible'. This is very important, since diagnosis and treatment of these conditions may significantly improve the person's life. Equally, if they are not detected, they can lead to further problems.

Depression

Depression in the elderly is surprisingly common and its incidence rises with age. Depression is not a function of ageing and it should always be treated seriously, as it puts people at risk of suicide.

- 15 per cent of over-65s suffer from depression.

- 30 per cent of over-75s suffer from depression.

- Only about 30 per cent of elderly sufferers of depression are known to their doctors; it is likely that this figure is so low because many of the people expect to have to put up with this as they get older.

KEY POINTS

- Depression is not a normal part of ageing.
- Depression puts people at risk of suicide.
- Males over the age of 75 have the highest suicide rates in most industrialised countries (although there is an increasing suicide rate among younger males in their 20s).
- In the elderly, depression is the most important predictor of suicide.
- Widowed elderly men have three times the risk of committing suicide as elderly men who are still married.

It is not always easy to tell if an elderly person is depressed, because they may seem to be quite content. Elderly sufferers from depression often do not complain about their depression, so relatives and friends may not be aware of it. People may put the person's irritability simply down to old age, when in fact they may be feeling miserable.

In the elderly, the classic symptoms of depression may be attributed to age and are therefore less likely to be questioned by the person and their family. There will probably be low mood and there may be an accompanying difficulty with thinking and concentrating. There may also be some disturbance of appetite and a tendency to wake early in the mornings. Sadness and tearfulness are obvious signs, but there may be more subtle signs, such as becoming more anxious or neglectful of oneself.

The following are indications of depression in the elderly:

- Sadness

- Fatigue

- Sleep difficulties

- Poor self-esteem

- Difficulty concentrating

- Memory problems

- Preoccupation with death and dying

- Suicidal thoughts

- Increased use of alcohol

- Loss of interest in hobbies

- Self-neglect

- Loss of appetite and weight loss

- Self-isolation.

It is common for a feeling of sadness or melancholy to be present when one is depressed, but it is not always apparent in the elderly. Indeed, sometimes the sufferer is not aware that they are depressed because they do not feel sad. Physical symptoms may be more dominant. They may feel that they can't be bothered with things, have a lack of motivation and energy, and simply attribute any physical symptoms to age. Yet they may also be depressed.

> ### KEY POINTS
>
> - Depression in the elderly may not always manifest itself as sadness or feeling down.
> - Treatment of the depression can make a huge difference to the person and improve their thinking as well as their mood.

Differentiating depression from dementia

Lowness of mood may not be present in dementia, but is more likely in depression (although not always, as mentioned above).

While elderly people with depression may feel apathetic and tend to withdraw, they will not experience the cognitive problems suffered by people with dementia.

Other emotions like guilt and poor self-esteem are common in depression, but not in dementia.

At its worst, thoughts of self-harm may be present in depression but are not present in dementia.

If the individual is orientated for time and place, that is, if they know who they are and who people around them are, and they know the time, date and year, they are probably not suffering from dementia.

In depression it is also common to have diurnal variation, which means a tendency to feel most depressed at the start of the day but gradually improving as the day goes on. This is not a feature of dementia, unless there is also depression.

Delirium

This is also referred to as an acute confusional state. It is characterised by confused thinking and disorientation; this may be for time and place in that the person is unsure if it is day or night, or where they are. The condition is another that is often confused with dementia, so it is important to investigate it; there may be another cause – such as chemical imbalance – caused by a urinary infection, a deficiency state or a problem with hormones – that can be treated with good results. On the other hand, the two can co-exist, though even if dementia is present, treating a toxic state should help.

KEY POINTS

- In delirium there is usually a clouding of consciousness. This means that the person usually feels sleepy or drowsy.
- Delirium usually occurs very quickly.

Delirium occurs in about 15–20 per cent of all general admissions to hospital,[10] so is very common when people are ill. The highest rates of delirium are in the elderly. The cause may or may not be obvious, but investigation is needed of any elderly person who suddenly seems to become confused, or experiences an alteration in consciousness, in that they become excessively sleepy or drowsy.

One of the commonest causes is actually due to medication. This is called iatrogenic delirium, which means 'doctor-made'. It comes from the Greek 'iatros', meaning 'doctor'. Some common causes of delirium are:

- Infections, especially urinary and respiratory

- Drugs – opiates, sedatives, anti-Parkinsonian drugs, anticonvulsants

- Metabolic problems –
  - low blood sugar
  - renal failure
  - liver failure
  - electrolyte imbalance of calcium, sodium and potassium.

- Alcohol excess

- Cardiovascular problems – silent heart attacks or mini-strokes (TIAs)

- Thyroid disease

- Nutritional problems – vitamin deficiencies, e.g. B12 or other vitamin B deficiency.

Hypothyroidism

This means an underactive thyroid. The condition used to be called myxoedema.

The thyroid gland is a butterfly-shaped gland in front of the windpipe in the neck. It produces thyroxine, a hormone that controls metabolism. If not enough thyroxine is being produced then the metabolism slows down and the patient develops hypothyroidism ('hypo' means low). Over a long time they may develop coarse skin, slow pulse, low energy, excess weight and mental and cognitive dulling.

KEY POINTS

- Hypothyroidism affects one in 50 women.
- Hypothyroidism affects about one in 1,000 men.
- Hypothyroidism increases the risk of heart disease, because it is associated with raised cholesterol levels.

In 1949 Dr Richard Asher of London first described a condition he called 'myxoedematous madness', which occurred in very rare instances when an extreme lack of thyroxine resulted in the patient developing hallucinations and psychotic symptoms. It is extremely rare these days, but in the elderly hypothyroidism can produce a confusional state or delirium that could be confused with dementia.

B12 deficiency

Vitamin B12 (cobalamin) is a key component in the metabolism of monoamines, which the body uses as neurotransmitters. Deficiency of this vitamin is associated with delirium and may even lead to a psychotic state, with wandering, hallucinations and delusions.

It is most likely to occur in the homeless, who may have diets lacking in nutrients. It can be reversed with injections of B12 and possibly folate. Recovery would be expected in days to weeks, with full recovery in about four weeks.

Parkinson's disease

This is a progressive neurological disorder that affects movement. It is caused by insufficient dopamine in parts of the brain called the basal ganglia. Dopamine is a neurotransmitter.

The condition tends to produce slowness of movement and a coarse tremor most marked at rest, which manifests as the classic 'pill-rolling' tremor, as if the person is rolling a pill between their fingers. It also can produce a mask-like or expressionless face, and a reduced ability to blink. It was first described by Dr James Parkinson in his medical paper 'An essay on the Shaking Palsy', now considered a classic of medical literature.

Depression is common in Parkinson's disease. This combined with the slowness of movement and expressionless face may make people think that the person with Parkinson's disease is not able to understand what others are saying and that their cognitive function is impaired.

KEY POINTS

- Parkinson's disease affects one in 500 people.
- It mainly affects people over the age of 50 years.
- There is no cure, but drugs can keep the condition under control.

As we saw in Chapter 6 (*Dementia with Lewy bodies and Parkinson's dementia*), two of the less common types of dementia can occur with Parkinson's disease. These are:

- Parkinson's disease dementia, when dementia occurs in someone who has had Parkinson's for some time.

- Dementia with Lewy bodies, when someone has had dementia first, or when they develop both dementia and Parkinson's disease at the same time.

Deafness

It is important to consider this, since if someone is unable to hear, the sensory isolation that it causes can lead to some confusion and this can in some instances be misinterpreted as meaning that the person is unable to understand what others are saying. Dementia can be misdiagnosed as a result.

Brain tumour

A tumour is the name for a growth of tissue. Correctly speaking it should be called a neoplasm, meaning 'new growth'. Tumours can be benign or malignant.

A benign tumour of the brain can cause symptoms that could be confused with dementia, by taking up space within the skull, thereby compressing the surrounding normal brain. Benign tumours do not spread elsewhere in the body.

Malignant tumours cause problems by spreading, either locally into surrounding tissues or by spreading through the bloodstream or lymphatic system to other parts of the body. It is possible to develop malignant brain tumours or to have secondary tumours that spread to the brain from other cancers, such as cancer of the lung. These are called metastases.

It is important to exclude possible tumours as a cause of symptoms in someone that is being investigated for dementia, because they could be treatable and indeed, may need to be treated as a matter of urgency.

CANCER AND DEMENTIA

Increasing age is a risk factor for dementia and also for cancer. One might expect that the two conditions would tend to co-exist. Rather surprisingly, rates of cancer are lower in people with dementia, and rates of dementia are lower in survivors of cancer.[11]

Charles Bonnet syndrome

Some people with sight loss experience visual hallucinations as a result. This can be very distressing to the individual, who may wonder whether they are developing dementia or a mental problem.

This condition, first described in the eighteenth century by the Swiss philosopher and scientist Charles Bonnet, seems to be a misinterpretation problem producing a false perception of what is seen. The person may think they have seen things or people who are not there. They can also see flashes, shapes, colours, faces, animals or eyes staring at them. It is most likely to occur if there is visual loss in both eyes. It occurs in about half of all people who have macular degeneration, a condition that affects the central part of the retina, causing difficulty seeing in the central part of the visual field.

Doing eye exercises may help. For more information see Macular Society in *Useful addresses* at the back of this book.

Mild cognitive impairment, MCI

Not all memory problems lead to dementia. Indeed, there is an important condition called mild cognitive impairment, which is characterised by difficulties in cognitive function, but which is not bad enough to be diagnosed as dementia.

Mild cognitive impairment, as the name implies, refers to difficulties with one or more of the cognitive or thinking functions of the brain. These problems can be with:

- Day-to-day memory

- Planning ability

- Language and communication

- Attention and concentration

- Visuospatial skills, or the ability to recognise shapes and assess distance between oneself and objects.

This is not a specific diagnosis, but a condition which may have different causes. It can be the first indication of Alzheimer's disease, vascular dementia, fronto-temporal dementia or Lewy body dementia, or it may be the result of other medical conditions, such as heart failure, diabetes or the side effects of drugs. It can also be the result of stress, anxiety or depression.

KEY POINTS

- Mild cognitive impairment is not a specific condition but has many causes.

- 5–20 per cent of elderly people will have MCI at some time.

- About 10–15 per cent of people with mild cognitive impairment will go on to develop dementia.

- Difficulties with memory could be an early sign of developing Alzheimer's disease.

- Difficulties with other cognitive functions could be an early sign of developing vascular dementia, fronto-temporal dementia or dementia with Lewy bodies.

THERE ARE DIFFERENT TYPES OF MEMORY

Memory is the name we give to the process of registering information, storing it and then recalling it. Broadly speaking there are two main types of memory, as we have seen earlier:

Short-term memory – for events of the day, names, addresses, messages and events of the recent past.

Long-term memory – the events of the more distant past, things that made an impact and things that were deliberately remembered.

In addition, we classify memory according to the sort of information that is stored. Here we have three types of memory:

Episodic memory – this is a memory tied to a specific time. That is, you remember things in episodes, as a soap opera on TV has episodes, so you remember things in a particular context. So, if the episode was about a restaurant, you might recall who you dined in that restaurant with.

Semantic memory – this is the memory of general facts, such as what a restaurant is, what a hospital is, what a hotel is.

Procedural memory – is about how to do things, for example, how to drive, use a cash dispenser, etc.

Difficulty with memory is the commonest of the cognitive abilities to be impaired. This makes up 66 per cent of cases of MCI. Others can have more of a problem with attention and concentration, for example, planning what to put on shopping lists. Still others may have trouble finding appropriate words.

It is important to establish whether MCI is present or not in order to determine whether further investigation is needed. This will involve referral to a memory clinic where a full assessment can be done.

The tests will include mental cognition tests which will look at memory, attention, decision making and judgement. This will show if there is dementia present, or whether it is so far only MCI. Subsequent visits will compare the mental cognition test results to determine whether there has been any deterioration, which would be consistent with a diagnosis of dementia, or whether any slight changes would be consistent with the normal ageing process of MCI.

The importance of MCI

You may wonder why it is important to find out if someone has MCI. You may think that it is part of normal ageing to be forgetful, since most people do experience some degree of forgetfulness as time goes on. However, in MCI it may not just be memory, but other cognitive functions, such as judgement or planning ability, that are affected.

The fact is that MCI does put people at risk of developing one of the dementias. If we can identify MCI, we can then reduce the risk of dementia and make life more pleasant for the individual.

The following things increase the risk of MCI:

• A family history of Alzheimer's disease and fronto-temporal dementia gives them a genetic predisposition.

- Smoking – increases the risk of arteriosclerosis, and therefore of hardening of the arteries and vascular dementia.

- Hypertension – high blood pressure increases the risk of arteriosclerosis and therefore of hardening of the arteries and vascular dementia.

- Alcohol – heavy drinking increases the risk of dementia, both Alzheimer's and alcohol-related dementia.

- Diabetes – having diabetes can double the risk of developing dementia.

- Obesity – increases the risk of arteriosclerosis and therefore of hardening of the arteries and vascular dementia.

We shall be looking at ways to reduce your risk of both MCI and dementia later in the book.

Part Two

DEALING WITH DEMENTIA

Use it or lose it

The phrase 'use it or lose it' intuitively makes sense: to retain an ability, you should keep doing it. Mental exercise, keeping yourself as mentally fit as possible, can help you to enjoy life.

My grandfather was a gardener until he was 88, when he decided to retire so that he could just look after his own garden. He used to say, 'It is better to wear out the hinges on a gate rather than leave them to rust.' That also seems to make sense. We know that physical exercise is good for the body in general. It is also good for the health of the brain, as it helps the general circulation.

As we saw in Chapter 3 (*What happens in dementia*), there are three stages, each of which may go on for several years. Life during the early and middle stages of dementia can certainly still be enjoyed by the individual, despite the progressive nature of the condition. So the person with dementia should be encouraged to keep doing familiar things, keep up hobbies and interests, with help where and when it is needed.

It is up to everyone else to be more accepting of dementia and to be more dementia-friendly, so that people with dementia can be included in communities and clubs and enabled to do normal things and live well with the condition.

Chapter 9

Getting the ball rolling – diagnosis

It is a sad fact that only one in three people with dementia sees a doctor and gets a diagnosis. Of those who do see a doctor, it is usually only after one or two years of struggling on with symptoms. This means that individuals are not receiving the best care that they can be given.

In 2012 the UK government announced the Prime Minister's Dementia Challenge to improve that figure and bring together the health service, social care, research, science and the charitable sector to transform how the country deals with dementia. The important message was that the government would increase funding of dementia research, increase awareness with a campaign encouraging people to visit the doctor if they are worried about having the condition, increase training and support, and provide funding for wards, care homes and housing for people with long-term conditions including dementia.

KEY POINTS

There are currently:

- More than 665,000 people diagnosed with dementia in England
- More than 86,000 people diagnosed with dementia in Scotland
- More than 18,000 people diagnosed with dementia in Northern Ireland
- More than 44,000 people diagnosed with dementia in Wales.
- It is estimated that there are currently at least 350,000 people with undiagnosed dementia, who are not accessing any support.

Getting a diagnosis

Part of the difficulty with getting a diagnosis is that so many people are unaware they have a problem. Their memory problems or other symptoms of mental decline are simply accepted by them and by people around them as things that are expected when one gets older. Also, people are often afraid to consider that dementia may be the reason, because there is still a stigma about it.

Cocktail chatter

One of the things that the person who is losing their short-term memory may do is to use cocktail chatter. That is, they simply use cues given by the person they are talking with to answer in a vague small-talk manner. They can seem to be lucid simply because they are responding and filling the air with words, albeit they are not listening and considering and replying in any constructive manner. They may seem quite happy to chatter like this and the people around feel reassured and see no reason for concern.

> **KEY POINTS**
>
> - Early diagnosis is important.
> - Assessment is a wider term than diagnosis, since it involves looking at how the condition is affecting the person's life and that of the family, and the strategies (or absence of them) used to help.

Early diagnosis

It is desirable to have a diagnosis made of dementia and of the type of dementia as early as possible. There are several reasons why:

- A diagnosis will explain why the person has been experiencing problems with their memory or other mental functions.

- It can be reassuring if dementia is excluded and a treatable reason is pinpointed.

- If dementia is diagnosed, it allows the person and the carers to understand the nature of the condition and the likely progression.

- If other conditions like depression are compounding the underlying dementia, treatment can make a big difference.

- It permits planning to be made and support to be mobilised.

- It may be that financial help can be put in place.

- It means that any treatment that can be given can be started soon.

There is no simple test that tells you conclusively whether dementia is or is not present. The first very important thing is for the doctor to sit and talk to the person and take a good history.

When should this first assessment be made?

As soon as any problem is seen to be affecting the person or their partner or family, an assessment should be made. So, if the person or members of the family are concerned, then that is an appropriate time to seek help, i.e. to make an appointment with the GP. The GP is the first point of contact with the health service for most people for most things, so there is a good chance that your doctor will already have some knowledge of the person and the person's family.

The GP will talk to the person and if possible to an accompanying friend or relative to get a good idea of the person's current state of health. A short mental health checklist, such as the Six Item Cognitive Impairment Test (6CIT), will probably be run through, which gives a good idea of how well oriented the person is in time, place and situation. In other words, do they know what time, date and time of the year it is, where they are and what they are doing.

It is likely that some basic blood tests will be arranged in order to exclude any of the treatable conditions that may mimic dementia. These include:

- Routine haematology to check haemoglobin, numbers of blood cells and ESR, a measure of inflammation

- Biochemistry tests – electrolytes (sodium and potassium), calcium, glucose and kidney and liver function tests

- Thyroid function tests

- Serum B12 and folate levels

- Possibly a urine test if the person seems confused, since a urinary infection can cause delirium.

- If the GP suspects a problem then a referral will be made to a local specialist. This may be at a specially designated memory assessment clinic or at the community mental health team, depending upon local organisation of the service.

KEY POINT

The levels of sodium and potassium, the body's electrolytes, are of crucial importance in the way that impulses are passed from neurone to neurone. Therefore electrolytes must be tested if someone is having memory problems.

THE SIX ITEM COGNITIVE IMPAIRMENT TEST

The original Six Item Cognitive Impairment Test (6CIT) was developed in 1983 in the USA. It was validated in the UK and altered in format in order to make it more user-friendly.[12] The 6CIT-Kingshill Version 2000© is the version used in the UK and is the test that your GP will be likely to use.

Six questions are asked and each answer is scored to produce a score out of 28.

1. What year is it?   [correct 0; incorrect 4]
2. What month is it?   [correct 0; incorrect 3]

A name and address is given and the person is asked to remember it.

3. What time is it, to the nearest hour? [correct 0; incorrect 3]
4. Count back from 20 to 1 [correct 0; 1 error 2, 2 or more errors 4]
5. Say the months of the year in reverse order
  [correct 0; 1 error 2, 2 or more errors 4]
6. The name and address is asked [correct 0; 1 error 2, 2 errors 4, 3 errors 6, 4 errors 8, all wrong 10]

Scores of: 0–7 are not significant;
  8–9 are probably significant;
  10–28 are highly significant.

The 6CIT-Kingshill Version 2000© is reproduced by permission of Dr Patrick Brooke. More information is available at www.6cit.co.uk.

The memory clinic

This is not just a clinic where one goes to get a diagnosis; it is a coordinating centre with a full range of assessment, diagnostic, therapeutic and rehabilitation services able to accommodate the different types and the different severities of dementia.

It works in partnership with local health, social care and voluntary organisations. Sometimes the memory clinic is a separate unit and sometimes it is part of the community mental health team. This depends upon local organisation of services.

Usually several visits to the memory clinic will be needed. The first visit will be an initial assessment. A second visit will be arranged for special investigations including a brain scan. A third visit is usually done to discuss the findings with the person, their family or their carer.

Not everyone is able to attend a memory clinic. It may be that the person is too infirm or incapacitated to attend, in which case a home assessment may be arranged with one or other members of the community mental health team. That may be a doctor or a psychiatric nurse.

Hospital specialists

Which sort of specialist sees the person depends upon their age and the symptoms that the person is experiencing, as well as the local organisation of services.

The following may be the first specialist to be seen:

- A psychiatrist specialising in the care of the elderly, sometimes referred to as a psychogeriatrician.

- A physician specialising in the care of the elderly, sometimes known as a geriatrician.

- A physician specialising in nervous diseases, known as a neurologist; this is most likely in the case of someone with early onset dementia.

- Any of the specialists may refer to another specialist if they feel it is necessary.

The following non-medical members of the team may also be asked to help in the assessment:

- An occupational therapist, who may assess the person at home or in the memory clinic or hospital. They will assess skills of daily living, the person's ability to prepare food and drink and their general ability to look after themselves. They may advise on adaptations or aids that may be helpful.

- A social worker, who can assess how well the individual's personal needs, interactions and finances are being met, and whether they need help in managing their affairs. This is important, since people with dementia are at risk of exploitation. It may be that the person with dementia will require residential care, possibly in a special residential home, or they may need help arranging attendance at dementia cafes or other venues.

- A psychologist, who may help in assessing the person's cognitive ability with various tests.

- A psychiatric nurse, who may have most to do with the person with dementia, seeing them regularly at home or in hospital.

The processes involved

The following things all form part of the process of information gathering and assessment that result in the diagnosis.

The medical history

This is taken by the doctor and rounded out by additional information and observations from a relative, carer or friend. In particular, questions will be asked about:

- Whether the person thinks they have any problems and, if so, what they are and how they are affecting their life. This is the most important question, since it gives an idea as to the person's insight into their condition.

- How things started to change, what were the first symptoms. Alzheimer's disease has a gradual onset and a steady progression. Vascular dementia often relates to a sudden onset and a jerky progression, worsening after each cardiovascular event (e.g. stroke or TIA).

- How the symptoms are affecting the person's life.

- The past medical history, looking at previous depression, head injury, medical conditions, operations and any medication they may be taking. This can be highly relevant, since some medication can cause confusion and can also make some dementias worse (e.g. drugs for Parkinsonism may worsen mental symptoms and cause hallucinations and delusions in patients with Lewy body dementia; equally, anti-psychotic drugs for hallucinations and delusions may further impair movement in these patients).

- The pre-morbid personality. This means the personality of the person before the symptoms started. Has there been a change in personality, as can occur in fronto-temporal dementia? Has the person become increasingly emotional, more aggressive, or emotionally blunted?

- The family history, since there may be a genetic tendency or a familial predisposition.

The physical examination

This is also performed by a doctor and is a general examination to determine the general state of health of the person and to diagnose any secondary conditions that may have a bearing on the person's state or that may improve their mental state (see Chapter 8, *Depression, delirium and mild cognitive impairment – things that can be confused with dementia*). A neurological examination is particularly important for determining whether there is any evidence of Parkinson's disease, brain tumour or another neurological condition.

In addition there will be blood tests, a chest x-ray if considered necessary, an electrocardiogram (ECG) to check heart function and an electroencephalogram (EEG) to check brainwave patterns. The EEG, which is not routine and will only be done if considered necessary, can help to determine if there is epilepsy or another physical brain condition, such as a tumour.

In rarer cases, when indicated, it may be necessary to do genetic testing for conditions like possible Huntington's disease.

- **The ECG** – The electrocardiogram is the name of the test used to record the electrical activity and the rhythm of the heart. It is sometimes also referred to as an electrocardiograph, but the common abbreviation of ECG is standard. The patient is connected to the machine by wires attached to electrodes that are strapped onto the limbs. Other wires are attached to the front of the chest and a recording is made. A reading is made on a long strip of paper by a hot-pen recorder. It is done with the patient fully conscious and causes no discomfort.

- **The EEG** – The electroencephalogram is a test used to measure the electrical activity from the various areas of the brain. Electrodes are placed over the scalp and a set of recorders show the activity as a series of squiggly lines on a screen. It is done with the patient fully conscious and does not cause any discomfort. It can be a very useful test if Creutzfeldt-Jakob disease is suspected, since very often the EEG shows characteristic periodic sharp spikes.

Mental state examination

This is a more specific assessment of the way the person is thinking. It may be done by the doctor as part of the first assessment. Mental state examination is done to indicate whether the person is depressed, anxious or experiencing any other mental illness. The testing will also discern whether the person is experiencing any hallucinations or delusions. A hallucination is an impression that something is present when in reality it is not. A delusion is a false belief in something that cannot be reasoned away (see Chapters 3 and 6 for further explanation).

The tests will also show if the person is filling in the gaps or making things up to cover gaps in their memory, a behaviour known as confabulating. And it will also look for evidence of getting in the loop, when the person continually repeats the same things after a few minutes, indicating problems with their short-term memory.

Cognitive examination

This may be done by the doctor but usually is done by a psychologist asking a set of formal questions that test various cognitive abilities. There are several of these tests, the most common one performed being the Mini-Mental State Examination (MMSE). This is marked out of a score of 30. A score of less than 24 is indicative of dementia.

The MMSE tests:

- Orientation in time and place – whether the person knows the time, date and where they are

- Attention and concentration

- Understanding

- Memory

- The ability to name things

- The ability to follow a three-stage instruction

- The ability to repeat a simple phrase

- The ability to copy a drawing

- The ability to understand a written statement

- The ability to write.

These tests can help to show what sort of problems the person is having. They also act as a baseline against which changes can be seen. This can help with diagnosis.

Brain scans

In the UK it is recommended by NICE, the National Institute for Health and Care Excellence, that a scan of the brain should be performed. These will pick up on haemorrhages, clots and tumours and give an idea about the volume of the brain and whether there has been any shrinkage in any specific parts or of the whole brain. There are three types of scan that may be arranged:

- *CT* – This stands for Computerised Tomography. X-rays of the brain are taken from various angles and analysed by a computer to build up a 3D image of the brain.

- *MRI* – This stands for Magnetic Resonance Imaging. It uses magnetism, ultrasound and computerised technology to build up multiple images of the inside of the body. These may show the tissues and any abnormalities in surprising detail. It can be an alarming investigation for people who are prone to claustrophobia, since with some scanners it necessitates being advanced through a large tunnel-like apparatus. This is the preferred type of scan if it is available, as suggested by NICE.

- *PET* – This stands for Positive Emission Tomography. It is an investigation that involves the injection of a radioactive substance that is taken up temporarily by cells in the brain. The scanner picks up on the radioactive emissions and looks at the flow of blood through the brain. It builds up a picture of the functional aspect of the brain. This is a highly sophisticated scan, which is performed less frequently than the CT scan or the MRI scan.

KEY POINTS

- An abnormal scan may help to diagnose dementia and point towards the type.
- A normal scan does not exclude dementia, since in the early stages of Alzheimer's disease the brain may show changes that are similar to ageing changes.

The diagnosis

Having assembled all the information from the patient, the history given by the patient and others, and added all of the results from the physical examination, blood and other tests, and the brain imaging, the doctor is in a position to come to a diagnosis.

Sometimes the doctor can only say that there seems to be a high probability that dementia is present. This might sound rather inexact. Indeed, the diagnosis is not always clean-cut. The cause and therefore type of the dementia may also be speculative rather than precise. As we have seen in part one of the book, there may be considerable overlap.

The discussion

This is the all-important part of the process, when the doctor sits down with the patient and relative, partner or carer and discusses the results. The person affected may or may not want to know the diagnosis, and this is important for the doctor to know.

On the other hand, for some people who have been struggling with their memory it may be a relief to know the reason. They may be relieved to know that it is, in fact, a brain disorder and not just getting old. For others, the thought of the word 'dementia' is so terrible that they may refuse to accept the diagnosis. They and their carer may try to insist that it is just age. Still others may have a severe emotional reaction to the diagnosis, believing it to be the end of their useful life. They may already be depressed and at risk of suicide and such news could tip them over the edge. The doctor and the team will have tried to elicit enough information about the person that they can gauge exactly how much the person and the carer need to know at this stage.

In the discussion the doctor will try to impart as clear an understanding as possible about the nature of the dementia and the course it is likely to take. It may be that the diagnosis is still unclear and that further information and tests will be needed. Often time will be part of that process, so that six months or a year down the line as the condition develops the diagnosis will become clearer.

It is highly important that the carer and the patient, if it is agreed to tell the patient, have some awareness of how the condition is likely to develop. This is so plans can be put into place for the future; that is, what practical things can help, what emotional help may be needed and what measures can be used to deal with finances and the person's affairs.

KEY POINTS

The aim of the discussion is to give the patient and the family or carer as much information as possible about the diagnosis and the nature of the dementia and how it may affect the person. All this is done taking into account the person's emotional state and the kind of effect the diagnosis may have on them.

It also aims to put in place measures that will allow the person to live well with dementia. The following measures are likely:

If drug treatment is thought to be helpful then it will be initiated.

Further appointments may be made to continue the discussion and to monitor progress.

Liaison with the GP is imperative, since the GP will still be the person's first point of contact.

A specialist nursing contact will be arranged.

A dementia adviser and local groups may be arranged.

A follow-up appointment may be made, probably for six months or a year ahead, depending upon the results of the assessment. At that time further cognitive tests are likely, to compare them with the first ones, so as to assess the person's condition and further needs.

Continuing contact and support

Receiving the diagnosis should not be the end of the process. Dementia is a progressive condition, so it is important to have some idea about the way the condition may affect the person and the family.

It may take time to come to terms with the diagnosis and so follow-up and ongoing contact with various people will be made. Who this is will depend on the organisation of local services.

General practitioner

The memory clinic will have been in contact with the GP, who will have their report on the diagnosis and the advised management plan. An appointment to see the person, either in the surgery or at home, will be made in order to discuss concerns and ensure that treatment, if any has been prescribed, is maintained.

Since confusion is likely to be an issue, it is important that drugs are monitored and given by a responsible person. That may be a member of the family, a carer or a member of staff if the person has been discharged to a residential home. The GP can liaise with the local pharmacist, who can arrange ongoing drug supplies, possibly delivery of the drugs to the home if needed, and can supply dosset boxes to help the individual if multiple drugs are to be taken at different times of the day. Dosset boxes have compartments, so that each day's supply is made up with compartments for the different times of the day. This enables the user or carer to ensure that the right drugs are taken at the right times.

At some stage it may be necessary to talk about driving. We will look at this further in Chapter 10 (*So I have dementia*).

Psychiatric nurse

The memory clinic may arrange for a psychiatric nurse to maintain contact. They will usually have extra experience with dementia care, so will be able to monitor changes in the person's mental health. They may liaise with both the GP and the memory clinic or the community mental health team. They can monitor medication and how the individual is responding to it. Any changes needed will be discussed with the GP.

Admiral Nurse

In some areas of the UK Admiral Nurses may be available. These are mental-health nurses who specialise in dementia. They generally work within the NHS and support people with dementia and their families. Some also work in residential care-home settings.

Admiral Nurses are named after Joseph Levy, who had vascular dementia and was known as 'the Admiral' because of his love of sailing. Dementia UK maintains the Admiral Nurse Academy, which trains Admiral Nurses. They are sometimes described as the Macmillan Nurses of dementia.

Services they can offer include:

- Skilled person-centred assessments of the needs of family, carers and individuals with dementia.

- Psychological support to help family, carers and people with dementia understand and deal with their feelings and emotions.

- Relevant information in the appropriate amount of detail and in a way that can easily be understood.

- Practical advice.

- Helping family and carers to develop and improve skills in care giving.

- Clear guidance about how appropriate services and sources of support can be accessed in local areas.

- Liaison with other professionals and organisations to ensure that families obtain coordinated support.

- Therapeutic, psycho-educational and social support groups for family carers.

- Referral to treatment and support services.

Dementia advisers

Alzheimer's Society, the oldest dementia charity in the UK, has an advisory service for people with dementia, their supporters and carers. The aim is to provide a named contact to help them cope with the ongoing condition. Referrals can be made via the memory clinic or sometimes through the GP, community mental health team or other health and social care professionals. The person or family can also make a direct request themselves.

The aims of the service are to:

- Provide information tailored to the individual's need

- Focus on the individual and empower them to access information

- Collaborate with other professionals.

The service includes an initial meeting at a centre or at the person's home to answer the person's questions, to arrange an information plan and to signpost services available, both nationally and locally.

A follow-up meeting two to four weeks later may answer any further questions and help with access to services and planning for the future. Regular meetings may be arranged within the information plan, including follow-up meetings with trained volunteers.

Dementia cafes

These are organised by the voluntary sector, including Alzheimer's Society and Age UK. They provide comfortable and supportive environments, a sort of cafe setting, for people with dementia and their carers to meet and socialise. Qualified staff and trained volunteers provide support and information, arranging talks and other activities.

One of the great problems that can occur when someone has dementia is that they become socially isolated. In part this can come about through apathy or because communication becomes more difficult. This can lead to depression, which in turn may compound the dementia. Maintaining social links and making new friends is good for people with dementia since it helps with self-esteem and keeps the sense of purpose that is so important for mental health.

Get a community care assessment

It is certainly worth getting a community care assessment, to which anyone with dementia is entitled. Sometimes called a needs assessment or a care assessment, it is done by the local authority social services department, though it does need a referral to be made. This can be done:

- By the GP, consultant or other health professional

- By the person with dementia, a relative or friend

- By a hospital social worker if the person is in hospital.

The aim is to assess the person's needs and put in place such measures and services as will help to meet those needs, including:

- Equipment and adaptations to the home

- Meals on wheels

- Home care, including help with cleaning and shopping

- Day care at a residential home, hospital unit or other venue

- Respite care.

An interview with the person with dementia and their carer will be arranged, generally with a social worker. The person with dementia has to be involved in the decision-making process, which is of the utmost importance, since it is about their needs.

The assessment by a named key social worker will look at the person's living arrangements, their general health and disabilities, their financial circumstances, and the person's worries and those of their carer. A questionnaire is likely to be needed. This is the self-assessment part of the process. If the person with dementia finds it too difficult then they will be helped. The assessment may be done at a single meeting, or it may be done over several meetings if the needs of the person are complex.

CARER'S ASSESSMENT

This is a separate assessment of the carer's needs. It is a good idea to request one and for that to be done alongside the needs assessment for the person with dementia. The aim is to ensure that if the carer is in education, or wishes to work, any help that is available should be accessed. They should effectively be able to have the same opportunities as a non-carer would have.

The care plan

After the assessment meeting the key worker will draw up a care plan. This should include:

- The needs that have been identified

- The desired outcomes and how they can be met

- A risk assessment

- A plan for dealing with emergency changes

- The result of the financial assessment

- The support that carers are willing and able to provide

- The support to be provided to meet the assessed needs

- The date that the plan will be reviewed.

There is no fee for the assessment, but the services provided may be charged for. This is done according to personal circumstances. The person may have to pay if they have sufficient means and savings, or they may be asked to provide a contribution. The charges have to be reasonable and the local authority will explain the way they have calculated the costings.

Advice on this can be obtained from the Citizens Advice Bureau or from Alzheimer's Society (see *Useful addresses* at the back of the book).

Personal budgets

Some authorities operate personal budgets rather than supplying services. This means that the person is given a direct payment in order to access the services themselves or through their family. This permits greater flexibility as the person can obtain services from the private or voluntary sectors.

KEY POINTS

- A community care assessment is provided free of charge by the local authority social services department in England and Wales.
- It is worth jotting down questions before the meeting.
- The meeting usually takes place in the person's own home.
- If it is done in hospital, then an adviser may visit the home to complete that part of the assessment of the person's needs.

Chapter 10

So I have dementia

Receiving the diagnosis that you have dementia can be a shock. It can take time to come to terms with the diagnosis, but there is still a lot that you can do to continue to enjoy life and live well with dementia.

Talk about it

Dementia is something that people have not wanted to talk about in the past. There is still a stigma about it, as I mentioned in the introduction. But it is gradually becoming less of a stigma as society is becoming more aware of and more concerned about helping people with dementia to live as full and enjoyable a life as possible.

It really does help to talk about your condition with friends and family. Tell them all you know and how you feel about it. This will help you come to terms with the diagnosis, to move on with your life and to plan for the future.

It is a good idea to think about who are the most important people to confide in. You might consider telling those people you are closest to. Also consider who is going to give you the most support.

You should talk to your doctor and to other professionals, such as an Admiral Nurse or a dementia adviser. Their knowledge can help you understand the condition, and their reassurance can also be extremely helpful.

If you have a condition that is going to progress, it is worth talking to family about your wishes as the disease advances. You can discuss with them the things you would like to do while you are able to enjoy doing them. Let family and friends know that you welcome them into your life, to share happy times with you. It is a good time to tell people how much they have meant to you and how much you still value their support and their love and friendship.

You may also want to talk about the care you will receive at the end of your life. This may upset family, but it is not being morbid to talk about such things; on the contrary, it is simply being practical. It is helpful for them to know what your wishes are regarding residential care and possibly hospital or hospice care in the last stage of dementia. That way there is not likely to be guilt or confusion in later years about what you would have wanted.

HOW TO TELL THOSE CLOSE TO YOU

The following may help:

- You don't have to tell them everything all at once. You can tell them when you are ready and you can tell them over more than one conversation.
- Be prepared to discuss the difficulties that may be experienced by you and your partner or relative as the condition worsens.
- From one of the dementia organisations or from your GP or the memory clinic get hold of some leaflets explaining the type of dementia that you have.

- Explain that you are still the same person; it is just that you have a progressive illness.
- Be prepared to accept help when it is offered. This can be good for you and for them.

QUESTIONS THAT YOU MAY WANT TO ASK YOUR DOCTOR

When you are first given a diagnosis of dementia it can be difficult to take it all in at once. The memory clinic will probably have given you some explanatory literature in the form of leaflets, but your GP is always a good person to ask about the condition. You can, of course, make an appointment at any time to discuss any concerns that you may still have.

The following are questions on which you may want some clarification:

- What type of dementia have I been diagnosed with?
- What does this mean?
- How is this likely to progress and over what time?
- How will that affect me?
- What resources are available which can help me live well with dementia and can help my family?
- What tests have been done and what do they show?
- What treatments are available to me?
- What side effects could there be?

Normal emotions to have

When the diagnosis is first received it is common to experience an emotional reaction. Indeed, you may experience several emotions. The thing to appreciate is that they are not uncommon; they are normal reactions and talking about them with friends, carers and professionals such as your doctor can be very helpful.

Denial

This is very common. The mind can find it hard to believe and so the diagnosis is denied. You may think that they have got it wrong, it could not possibly happen to you. This usually changes and acceptance comes. It may be the enormity of the diagnosis, but as with bereavement, when it just seems too hard to accept that a loved one has gone, time will soften the emotion and with that will come acceptance.

Anger

It is common to be angry that this has happened, since it suddenly changes your life, your plans for the future. Again, this will tend to soften over time, especially if you talk about it. And the plans you made can still happen; they may simply need to be modified as time goes on.

Relief

For many people it is actually a relief to be given a diagnosis for the symptoms that they may have been experiencing for some time. There is now a reason for them, and with that explanation you may find that the anxiety you were feeling will begin to ease.

Anxiety

On the other hand, sometimes the diagnosis can be the cause of anxiety. This can be anxiety about yourself, about the future, or about others. How, for example, will it affect your partner, if you are already a carer for them? Or how will it affect your finances, your ability to drive, and so forth. Again, talking about this will help to get things in proportion. Your doctor may be able to help with strategies that you can use to feel less anxious.

Isolation

You may feel isolated by the diagnosis. It may seem that no one understands what you are going through.

Depression

This can occur in conjunction with dementia, or it can occur as a reaction to the diagnosis. Talking about feeling sad with family can help, and if it persists you can talk to your doctor. Having depression treated can improve how you feel and may also help the other difficulties you have been experiencing with memory and thinking.

Guilt

Some people feel guilty about having a condition that may put a strain on relationships or make them more dependent on others. There is no need for guilt; it is an emotion which will only make you feel worse. Talking about how you are feeling with your loved ones is worth doing. Their reassurance will often do a lot to make you feel better. The simple act of talking about it may have an effect on its own, because you are getting it off your chest.

If you find that you are troubled with an emotion for several weeks and it won't go, then see your doctor. It may be that you are suffering with anxiety or depression (see Chapter 8, *Depression, delirium and mild cognitive impairment – things that can be confused with dementia*).

Be proud of who you are

Although you are living with dementia, it is also worth making your mark. You will have had a lifetime of valuable experiences, and these will be worth celebrating. You could, for example, volunteer to speak to people newly diagnosed with dementia, so that they can see how life can still have meaning. You could suggest this to your doctor or you could join one of the dementia organisations listed in *Useful addresses* at the end of the book.

You could write letters to your children or your grandchildren, expressing how much you love them. Tell them about your life and how things have changed. It is an opportunity to put these things down on paper for them to read at a point in the future when perhaps you no longer feel like writing.

Coping with memory problems

Difficulty with memory is characteristic of dementia and is often the first thing that persuades someone to seek help. The following strategies may help you to deal with failing memory:

- Avoid getting tired – if the brain is tired, it affects your memory.

- Keep a diary – a record of what you have done each day will be useful and writing it helps the cognitive process of thinking and composing your thoughts.

- Have a memory hub – that is, have a central place in the home, perhaps a dining room table or a desk, where you can keep important notes and put things that you want to be able to find quickly. Rather than having everything scattered about the home, get into the habit of having one place for car keys, house keys, the dosset box for the drugs you take, your purse.

- Keep a whiteboard in the kitchen – to record your timetable for the week and things that you have to do.

- Label doors, drawers, cupboards and cabinets.

- Have a list beside the telephone of people that you may need to call – GP and other care professionals, carers, family and reliable friends.

- Order a daily newspaper – this helps to keep you aware of what is happening in the world. It also tells you the date.

- Tell your family that you are happy about being gently reminded to do things and about things that seem to slip your memory.

- When showering or having a bath, so that you don't forget whether you have washed your hair, have a routine. For example, move the conditioner and shampoo from one side of the shower or bath to the other once you have used them.

- Use your photograph album to remind you of the things that have happened in your life, and who people are.

- Make a deal with your carer that you will both do whatever you can to encourage your memory.

We will look at things that your partner or carer can do to help in the next chapter.

Things you can do to help yourself

Avoid bad habits

We touched on this in the chapter on reducing your risk of dementia. The same advice holds true if you have dementia. The fewer pollutants you take into your system the better.

Avoid smoking.

Do not overuse alcohol.

Do not use alcohol to help you sleep – it is actually counter-productive and tends to make you wake in the night.

Avoid fast food, since this can promote inflammation, which may make dementia worse.

Look after your physical health

Staying as physically well as you can will help you to live well with dementia.

- Have regular health checks with your doctor.

- Get into a regular routine and build in some exercise. That doesn't have to mean strenuous exercise, but simply some form of regular exercise. If you are up to it, then swimming, golf and sports such as tennis are good for cardiovascular health. Walking, gardening and housework are all beneficial. Aim to include some exercise in your daily routine.

- Eat healthily and aim to have regular meals, the less processed food the better. The Mediterranean type of diet seems to be the most beneficial in helping dementia, since it is the best in maintaining the general health of the circulation.

Learn to relax

Being stressed seems to interfere with mental processes like thinking, concentrating and making decisions.

The following are useful to help you relax:

- Music – the poet and playwright William Congreve wrote in 1697 that 'music has charms to soothe a savage breast'. It was true all those centuries ago and it is still true today. Listening to your favourite type of music is a useful way of relaxing.

- Watching a favourite television programme or listening to a regular radio show that interests you.

- Smelling the flowers, watering plants and spending time in the garden. A review of 17 studies showed that these activities can soothe the anxiety of some people with dementia.[13]

- Painting and enjoying art.

- Enjoying things that make you laugh. Humour can be a great aid to relaxation.

- Doing group activities such as dancing, yoga or meditation.

- Progressive muscle relaxation. This is a useful technique for relaxing, which I will cover in Chapter 14 (*Using the Life Cycle to help cope with dementia*).

Try to stay positive

The diagnosis of dementia takes time to accept, but it is not a death sentence. Dementia can be lived with for many years, so the person with dementia, friends and family should strive to cherish their time together. We will look at ways to stay positive in Chapter 14 (*Using the Life Cycle to help cope with dementia*).

Maintain your independence but accept help

Many people with dementia want above all else to maintain their independence. They want to manage their own affairs and to stay in their own home. That is certainly possible, at least in the early stages of the condition.

One of the problems with dementia, of course, is its progressive tendency to affect communication and drive. The person may start to isolate themselves from family and friends. This can start because you may not feel bothered about maintaining relationships, or you may not want to join in conversations. This is something you should strive to avoid. Instead, try to keep up with relationships and try to join in conversations; isolation may make you feel worse rather than better.

To help you to live independently you should try to build and maintain a strong support network. The more help you can get to stay independent, the better. The message is not to refuse it.

Help can come from:

• Your GP and other health professionals.

- Family and friends – so keep regular contact and make sure you have help with shopping, meals and social life.

- Social services – who can arrange:
  - domestic help
  - personal care to help with washing, dressing and going out
  - day care to meet other people.
- Voluntary agencies – such as Alzheimer's Society, Age Concern and British Red Cross, which offer information, day care, dementia cafes, drop-in centres and befriending schemes.

Work

If you are still working when you have been given the diagnosis of dementia, you may feel that you should stop working. That should not be an automatic decision, since work may be good for you as long as you are still coping with it. There are, after all, many reasons why people work, apart from the financial reward of a pay packet or salary. Work may enhance your self-esteem and may provide you with mental and social stimulation.

So don't automatically stop work. Talk about it with your employer and you may be pleasantly surprised to find that they are happy for you to continue. Or it may be possible to reduce your hours. The situation can be observed as you go along. Another possibility may be to accept a different, less stressful role at work.

On the other hand, you may decide that you want to stop work, in which case do check up on any benefits you may be entitled to. And you may be eligible to draw your pension (see below).

Driving

You are actually obliged to inform the Driver and Vehicle Licensing Agency (DVLA) and your insurance agency once you have been diagnosed with dementia. This does not mean that you will automatically lose your licence, but your case will be assessed. You should stop driving while they make their decision. They will probably seek a report from a doctor and you may be asked to take a driving test.

If you hold a Heavy Goods Vehicle (HGV) licence or a Public Carriage Vehicle (PCV) licence, then you will not be allowed to keep it.

It is important to be aware that dementia is progressive, so judgement and decision making will become less certain. The person with dementia has a responsibility to be safe, as does every driver, so it may be a sensible decision to stop driving.

Sex

A person with dementia may have a normal sex life in the early stages of the condition. As it progresses there is likely to be a loss of libido. Some people lose the libido early on, which may be distressing to their partner. If this is the case, it is worth talking about it with your doctor or Admiral Nurse. There may be strategies that you can try to stimulate renewed interest; for example, trying to create a romantic mood, showing affection and love. Your doctor will discuss whether any drug treatment would be appropriate.

On the other hand, some people as part of the disinhibition that occurs in dementia may experience an increased libido. This may become inappropriate and may have to be considered as a behavioural problem. Again, it is worth talking this over with the doctor, since there may be drug treatment that will reduce the libido.

Get organised

Handling your affairs may already be proving difficult. As the condition progresses it will certainly become harder, so it is a good idea to put measures in place.

Day-to-day bills

Talk with your family and your carer about your normal bills. It is worth sitting down and reviewing all of the bills that need regular payments.

The following are worth considering:

- Setting up direct debits or standing orders with your bank to pay utility bills, e.g. gas, electricity, telephone.

- Opening a joint account with a partner or spouse, so that they can pay bills on your behalf.

- Getting a chip and signature bank card instead of a bank card with a PIN number, if you have difficulty remembering numbers. You need only sign a receipt instead.

- A third-party mandate allows a named person, usually a carer, to have access to your bank account. Your bank can advise on this.

- Have any benefits you are entitled to paid directly:
    - into a post office card account
    - into a bank or building society account.

- A second person can be nominated as a 'permanent agent' to access the post office card account, as long as you are able to consent.

Benefits

You may be entitled to receive benefits. A social worker or Citizens Advice Bureau adviser may be able to help you with this (see *Useful addresses* at the back of the book). A person with dementia may be eligible for Attendance Allowance (AA) and Personal Independence Payment (PIP). They are not automatic, but have to be individually assessed. The following conditions apply to these payments:

- They are tax-free.

- They are independent of National Insurance contributions.

- They are independent of personal savings.

- A medical examination is usually required.

- The person is still allowed to work.

To apply for these benefits, go to the Department for Work and Pensions (DWP) website, which gives information on each benefit and on how to claim. If you cannot manage to access this yourself, then ask a relative or your carer.

Attendance Allowance

If you are over 65 years of age, you may be eligible to receive Attendance Allowance. To be eligible you have to demonstrate difficulty in looking after yourself in areas such as washing and bathing, dressing, eating and going to the toilet.

Attendance Allowance is paid at two different rates; how much you get depends on the level of care that you need because of your disability. The lower rate is for frequent help or constant supervision during the day, or supervision at night. The higher rate is for help or supervision throughout both day and night.

The other benefits you get may increase if you get Attendance Allowance.

Personal Independence Payment

This benefit replaced Disability Living Allowance in 2013. Personal Independence Payment (PIP) helps with some of the extra costs caused by long-term ill-health or a disability if you're aged 16 to 64. There are two rates depending on how your condition affects you, not the diagnosis of the condition itself.

You'll need an assessment to work out the level of help you get. Your award will be regularly reassessed to make sure you're getting the right support.

State pension

A taxable state pension is paid to people who have made sufficient National Insurance contributions. The state pension age for men is currently 65. The state pension age for women born on or before 5 April 1950 is 60. The pension age for men and women is gradually rising and after 2020 will be 68 for both men and women.

It is worth discussing with your social worker or the Citizens Advice Bureau to see whether you are eligible for any other benefits. Pension Credit may be available if you are unable to claim state pension, and Income Support may be available if you are below pension age.

Planning for the future

This is very important, because there will probably come a time when you are not able to make decisions.

Make a will

This is something that many people never think of doing, but it is a very good idea to make a will. If you die without making a will (known as dying intestate), then it can take a long time to sort out your estate. Also, it may be that you would wish to leave your assets or particular possessions to certain people. If you have made a will, then this will be straightforward. If not it may cause problems for your family after you die.

To make a will, simply see your solicitor, who will draw it up according to your wishes. In order to make the will you have to have 'testamentary capacity'. This means that you have to be capable of making your own decisions at that time. In the early stages of dementia you may still be able to do this.

The Mental Capacity Act of 2005

This sets out a statutory framework to empower and protect people who may lack capacity to make some decisions for themselves. It makes clear who can take decisions in which situations, and how they should go about this.

Anyone who works with or cares for an adult who lacks capacity must comply with the MCA when making decisions or acting for that person. This applies whether decisions are life-changing events or more everyday matters and is relevant to adults of any age, regardless of when they lost capacity.

The underlying philosophy of the Mental Capacity Act is to ensure that those who lack capacity are empowered to make as many decisions for themselves as possible and that any decision made, or action taken, on their behalf is made in their best interests.

The five key principles in the act are:

- Every adult has the right to make his or her own decisions and must be assumed to have capacity to make them unless it is proved otherwise.

- A person must be given all practicable help before anyone treats them as not being able to make their own decisions.

- Just because an individual makes what might be seen as an unwise decision, they should not be treated as lacking capacity to make that decision.

- Anything done or any decision made on behalf of a person who lacks capacity must be done in their best interests.

- Anything done for or on behalf of a person who lacks capacity should be the least restrictive of their basic rights and freedoms.

Lasting power of attorney (LPA)

This is a legal document that you can sign, providing you have the mental capacity to do so. Again, it can be made in the early stages of dementia. It allows you to choose someone who can make decisions for you about your health or your welfare, as well as financial decisions if you are unable to make those decisions yourself.

There are two types of lasting power of attorney:

- *Financial LPA*, which gives the attorney (the person named to make the decisions on your behalf) the power to make decisions about your financial and property matters, such as selling a house or managing a bank account.

- *Welfare LPA*, which gives the attorney the power to make decisions about your health and personal welfare, such as day-to-day care, medical treatment, or where you should live.

Advance decision or living will

Many people want to make their wishes known about treatment that they would like to refuse should they be unable to communicate in the future. This is commonly called a living will, but the name is in fact a bit misleading, since it has nothing to do with money or property, as a will does. More correctly it is called an 'advance decision'.

Under ordinary circumstances when you fall ill there will be an opportunity to discuss treatment with your doctor. If, however, you are suddenly taken ill and admitted to hospital when unconscious, and are therefore unable to communicate your wishes, then the medical team will try to use all possible means to save your life. If this is not what you would wish – for example, if you had a stroke and were unable to communicate – then you might consider making an advance decision.

This is a notification on paper that in certain circumstances you would wish to refuse certain types of treatment. These could include resuscitation or perhaps a desire not to be given intravenous drugs, a blood transfusion or parenteral feeding (feeding through a drip into a vein).

An advance directive is legally binding in England and Wales. Medical and nursing professionals must accept your decision regardless of their own opinions. It cannot be revoked by the family. The situation is different in Scotland and Northern Ireland.

Sometimes the term 'advance statement' is used, but this is not quite the same thing. Whereas the advance decision is a refusal of treatment, an advance statement is an expression of the individual's desires. It may relate to food preferences and religious or philosophical beliefs. It is not legally binding.

KEY POINTS

- An advance decision is notification of a refusal to have treatment, should the individual be unable to communicate with medical professionals.

- An advance decision can be made by anyone over the age of 18 who is of sound mind.

- It is a legal document that cannot be overruled by the family or medical or nursing staff.

- The individual who makes it can revoke it at any time.

- Doctors and family should be aware that an advance decision has been made.

Organ donation

The person with dementia can still donate their organs after they die. There is no age limit; the physical condition of the organs is the deciding factor. Specialist professionals make the decision in each case which organs and tissues are suitable, and organs from people in their seventies and eighties can still be used. All donors have the choice of which organs and tissues they wish to donate.

The NHS Organ Donor Register is a confidential national database that holds details of more than 20 million people who have made the decision to donate organs (see *Useful addresses* at the back of the book).

Brain donation

You may wish to donate your brain to scientific research after death. The brains of people with and without dementia are invaluable for scientific research into the causes of these conditions. Researchers need brains from people with any form of dementia and any stage of the condition. As mentioned earlier, many people die from other causes, such as heart attacks, stroke or pneumonia in the early and middle stages, rather than directly from dementia.

Making a decision to donate your brain after your death can give some satisfaction, since studying your brain may lead scientists to the breakthrough that is needed to change our understanding and treatment of the disease, a contribution to science that may be of inestimable value to future generations.

For more information on this, contact Brains for Dementia Research Coordinating Centre (see *Useful addresses*).

Chapter 11

Caring for someone with dementia

Caring for someone with dementia can be a frustrating, harrowing and distressing process. It can go on for several years, during which time it may seem that the personality of the loved one gradually disappears. It is important for carers to be prepared for the changes that will occur and not to allow what may be a difficult situation to make them feel ill.

Remember that the person with dementia is not becoming another person. They are still the person you admired, loved and had fun with. They have a disease that is making them forgetful and affecting the way that they think and behave.

At some points you will have to make decisions based on the person with dementia's individual personality. For example, you may decide that it is worth going on holiday because, even though initially it could be confusing for the person with dementia, it could also be a happy time and a way for them to live well. Indeed, there is much that you can do to enable them to live well with dementia, and to enable you, the carer, to enjoy your own life and feel proud of caring for the person with dementia.

You are not alone

That is the first thing to appreciate: you are not the only person caring for someone with dementia. This means that there are lots of people who have experienced what it is like, and you can meet them and gain from their experience in local groups, dementia cafes and also in support agencies on the internet. There are several useful addresses to be found at the back of the book.

But the message is, don't expect yourself to soldier on alone. There is help available as long as you access it.

DEMENTIA FRIENDS

This is an Alzheimer's Society initiative. People with dementia get by with a little help from their friends, so they need friends.

Anybody can become a Dementia Friend. It means understanding a bit more about dementia and the small things you can do to help people with the condition. This could be helping someone find the right bus or being patient in a checkout queue if someone with dementia is taking longer to pay.

People with dementia want to live well and to be able to carry on going about their daily lives and feeling included in their local community, but they sometimes need a helping hand to do so. Dementia Friends learn a little bit about what it's like to live with dementia and turn that understanding into action.

Being a Dementia Friend isn't about volunteering, but it is about being a friend and being helpful to people with dementia. Take a look at the Dementia Friends website for details (see *Useful addresses*).

Effective communication

Learning how to communicate effectively with the person with dementia is extremely important. The person with dementia has a condition that is gradually going to worsen, and parts of their brain that control understanding, thought processing and language ability are deteriorating. They will lose their ability to understand subtle nuances, so they may not understand jokes and humour. They may get frustrated at their inability to think of words, or cross when they cannot express themselves. They may get in the loop, where they continually ask the same question no matter how often they are given a response.

There are several strategies you can learn to use to aid communication:

- When you talk to them, always try to engage eye contact.

- Speak clearly so that they can hear you.

- Speak calmly, and never allow yourself to get cross or show frustration as this may distress them.

- Ask them if they would like you to find words for them if they are having difficulty.

- Try to get into their mind and empathise with how they are thinking at whatever stage of their illness they are in.

- Be careful about asking questions that they will be unable to process. For example, if they are crying, don't quiz them about what is the matter. They may not know or be able to verbalise it. Instead, perhaps say, 'You seem to be upset; let's think how we can make you feel better.'

- Be careful about asking why they have done things that seem to be incorrect. If they have put crockery in the washing machine or clothes in a food cupboard, don't castigate them. It is far better to say, 'You seem to have put the crockery in the washing machine. Did you mean to put it in the dishwasher?' And then show them by taking it out and putting it in the proper place.

- Be aware that the body language of the person with dementia may tell you things about how they are feeling. Try to pick up on this. For example, repetitive movements may indicate that they are feeling anxious and scared; withdrawing may indicate that they feel overwhelmed.

- Use your own body language to help communicate. For example, use hand movements to indicate directions or to illustrate some activity that they may want to do.

Early stage care

You may care to refresh your memory as to what to expect by looking at Chapter 3 (*What happens in dementia*). But broadly, in this stage there may be only minimal disturbance. The person may have memory problems and difficulty in concentrating or making decisions, yet other people may not be aware that they have a problem.

This early stage can continue for several years, so the person with dementia can still lead a useful and enjoyable life.

What you can do to help

Your main role at this time is to be supportive. Aim to maintain their self-esteem, their sense of well-being, their mood and their independence.

Routine

Establishing a routine is a good idea. People with dementia generally like routines as it tends to keep them orientated. Try to establish:

- Regular sleep patterns with bed times and rising times

- Regular drug-taking times

- Regular meals

- Social times

- Shopping days

- Time to have fun with activities or TV or radio.

Keep yourself up to date with dementia news

Join one of the support organisations and keep up to date on anything new that can be applied to the life of the person with dementia, if it seems helpful. In that regard, attending a support group or a dementia cafe together may be helpful for both of you.

Jog their memory

Memory difficulties at this stage tend to be relatively easy to cope with, and you may just need to jog their memory about such things as:

- Appointments

- Remembering people's names and faces

- Finding the right word

- How to do things, e.g. making meals, drinks, operating household gadgets

- Taking medication

- Taking meals.

Planning and organising

This will probably prove more difficult as the condition progresses. You should try to help the person with dementia rather than just take over. Enabling them to stay independent is more likely to maintain their sense of worth and self-esteem than doing everything, which will make them dependent, even if sometimes it may seem easier just to do things yourself. Helping them arrange a shopping trip and make a shopping list for themselves encourages them to use the appropriate thought processes.

It is often helpful to work with the person with dementia as if you are a team trying to formulate a plan. For example, with any task discuss how you can break it down into simple parts that are easy to do. Then the task can be accomplished more easily. Making a meal is a good example of where this task approach will be helpful to the person with dementia.

Plan for the future

This can be difficult to talk about, but it is the right time to put in place all the financial and legal measures that can only be done while the person has the mental capacity to do so. So talk about managing money, making a will, considering advance decision and power of attorney (see Chapter 10, *So I have dementia*). For the same reason, it is also the time to talk about driving and safety issues for the future.

It may also be the time to talk about the person's wishes for end-of-life care, their wishes regarding a funeral and their wishes for a burial or cremation; if you leave it too late, you may never know what their wishes were. Obviously this can be an upsetting discussion, so make sure to do so at a time when the person with dementia seems happy to discuss it. It can be broached opportunistically: if a time arises when someone they know dies, ask what they would wish for – a cremation or burial – when the time comes.

Support their emotional needs

The person with dementia may experience all manner of emotions. They may feel depressed, anxious, frustrated, cross or guilty. They may have difficulty in expressing those emotions. You can help by:

- Encouraging them to talk about their feelings.

- Keeping them involved in activities and hobbies.

- Ensuring that they do not become isolated.

Enjoy being together

If you live with the person with dementia, remember to have fun together. Enjoy this time. It will not be difficult all the time. Indeed, you will probably notice that it is a fluctuating course, in that some days will be good and other days may be less so. It is very much about living well with dementia.

Reminiscence book and box

In the early stage of dementia it is a good idea to begin a reminiscence book: an album of photographs from the person's life in chronological order. Many people have photographs tucked away in various places, but having them all together can be helpful to the memory. It can be a fun thing for the carer and the person with dementia to do together. You can also put in pictures of things that are associated with that time. It is a good idea to annotate the album with dates and snippets of information, in addition to which you can also have a reminiscence box containing objects that have a story in the person's life.

These resources can be brought out and used to jog the memory. They probably have happy associations which can help to calm someone down and distract them if they are getting distressed when they are in the middle stage; and they can also be of use in the late stage, because the person may still be able to understand more than is apparent.

The person with dementia can be asked to tell the story behind a picture or object, and just enjoy reminiscing. However, some photographs may trigger upsetting memories – for example, seeing photographs of a former partner – so it is as well to be aware that this may happen.

Middle stage care

This stage is usually the longest and can last for several years. It can be very challenging for a single carer. More care is going to be needed and this will probably mean accessing more help for you as a carer.

The main difficulties that people experience in this stage relate to communication, where the person with dementia may have real problems expressing their thoughts and emotions. They may want to talk or be talked to, which the carer may find draining. If the carer is reluctant to engage in this conversation or doesn't seem to have time, then the person with dementia may become irritable or grumpy. This is where the way that you communicate with the person with dementia and understand their body language becomes very important.

Difficulty with concentration is another big problem. Things that the person enjoyed in the past may seem too difficult, so they may want to be entertained by the carer rather than playing a game or doing a task themselves.

They may have problems with simple tasks, such as dressing, making drinks and food, and managing money and affairs. Their behaviour may be erratic and some people may have hallucinations and delusions.

It is not all gloom, however. As with the early stage, it will be a fluctuating course and there will be good days as well as not so good ones.

Be patient

This is one of the main attributes that needs to be cultivated. The actions and the attitude of the person with dementia may be very variable and erratic. Their brain will be undergoing change and they may well get frustrated at not being able to do things. They may seem obstinate and refuse to do things that you want them to. That obstinacy may be the only way that they are able to show their frustration.

Routine

As with the early stage routine is good, and so it is useful to try to maintain the same routine, though be prepared to modify it.

On some days the person with dementia may not want to get dressed, have a bath or sit down at a certain time. When this happens, be flexible and accommodating. Reason with the person but don't coerce them into doing things.

If they don't want to take a bath, then leave it for the time being and come back to the matter later on, when the person with dementia is more settled. Suggest then in a cheerful and encouraging manner that it would be an enjoyable thing to have a nice, relaxing bath to feel fresh and clean before doing something else.

Changing behaviour

The alterations in people's behaviour can be the hardest thing to cope with for the carer and the family. The following can occur:

- Depression

- Anxiety and agitation

- Anger and aggression

- Clinginess

- Repetitive behaviour

- Irritability

- Paranoia and suspiciousness

- Disinhibition

- Wandering

- Sleep problems.

If these changes are sudden and sustained it may be that there is a physical reason, so do not simply assume that it is a result of the dementia. Have a doctor check the person, because there may be a treatable cause.

Depression

As mentioned in Chapter 8 (*Depression, delirium and mild cognitive impairment*), low mood is not always a feature of depression in the person with dementia. They may seem more apathetic and reluctant to do things. If you suspect depression then contact your doctor, since treating it can make a big difference.

Anxiety

This is not uncommon and is perfectly understandable. The person with dementia may be finding the world a very frightening place. Even the familiar home may seem strange. It can help to have an awareness of the following potential causes of anxiety:

- Change of residence, perhaps moving to a residential home

- Change in the environment, such as travelling or having to go into hospital

- Having more people around than normal, such as when family or guests arrive

- Changes of carers

- Noise

- Drug side effects

- Too much caffeine from coffee or tea

- Alcohol.

Try to make the person's surroundings as comfortable and relaxing as possible. Music may help, as may pleasant smells, pictures and familiar personal possessions. Try to eliminate the triggers and keep the environment calm. Distraction is often very helpful, in that it takes their mind off the moment and the thoughts that they are having at the time so as to focus instead on something more pleasant that doesn't cause them anxiety. For example, music may be a good distraction.

Anger and aggression

This can take the form of physical or verbal aggression. It may seem totally out of character, which makes it even more difficult to accept. However, this is where patience comes in. The carer has to remain patient and calm, for that in itself can have a calming effect on an angry person.

It's important to appreciate that the condition itself is what makes the person angry; the person is not behaving aggressively on purpose. It is also important to be aware of potential triggers, such as the following:

- Physical reason – the person may be in pain but not be able to communicate it or explain its possible cause. This may be a number of things including:

  - urinary infection
  - chest infection
  - stroke
  - silent heart attack.

- Medication side effects – has there been a recent alteration in the drugs?

- Has the person had enough sleep?

TIPS FOR DEALING WITH AGGRESSION

- Try to identify the cause.
- Is there a legitimate reason for anger? Have you done something to upset them?
- Rule out pain or other physical discomfort. This may mean obtaining a medical opinion.
- Focus on the feeling rather than on what the person says, if they are being abusive. That is, don't take what they are saying personally, but look for a way of calming the anger.
- Do not react yourself, but stay calm.
- Speak reassuringly and in a calm manner.
- Use music or a calming activity such as massage or stroking their hands or brushing their hair.
- Do something different to distract the person from the moment and from their anger.
- Do not coerce or use force in any way.
- Make sure that the person cannot injure him or herself.
- Do not put yourself in danger, if necessary moving back and waiting for calmness to return.

Clinginess

Some people with dementia become very clingy and do not allow their carer to be out of vision. They are usually staying close because of fear. This can be a result of two early psychological reflexes that develop in toddlers. The first is the mother-withdrawal reflex, where a young toddler will cry when the mother moves away because mother is provider and protector. The second is the stranger-approach reflex, which induces crying and distress when a stranger approaches, because the toddler perceives them as a threat. As the dementia progressively affects the person's brain there is a loss of neurones, and old reflexes like this, which had been suppressed by more complex neural pathways, can resurface.

Clinginess can be very wearing on the carer. One way of reducing this is to try diluting the contact. In other words, try introducing other carers for short periods. Also having respite care to give the carer a break may lessen the clinginess.

Repetitive behaviour

This is the loop phenomenon I talked about earlier in the book. The person seems to get a question or thought stuck in their mind and will ask the same question over and over again, despite it having been answered. Or it can take the form of repeating an activity indefinitely. They may pace the floor, or repeatedly open and close a door.

Fear again seems to be part of the problem. Remember that the world can seem a frightening place to the person with dementia. The repetition may be to do with comfort and security. They may find it reassuring to get the answer, albeit only transiently.

TIPS FOR DEALING WITH THE LOOP PHENOMENON

- What is the trigger? Is it in certain circumstances or when certain people are around? Is it at a particular time? If you can pinpoint the trigger you may reduce the repeated question or activity.

- What emotion does the person seem to be experiencing? If you can deal with that emotion then the loop may be broken.

- It may be possible to turn a repeated action into a useful activity. If someone is tapping or patting the arm of a chair, suggest that they do something like dusting. Give them a duster and make the dusting movement to show what you mean.

- For repeated questioning, try giving a written answer. If the question is about time or date, indicate a clock or a calendar. This encourages them to read or to tell the time themselves.

- Don't ignore repeated questions, but give the answer and be patient. It will eventually settle.

- Repeated actions may actually be helping the person to reduce their anxiety. They don't have to be stopped. And they don't have to be stopped just because the carer finds them irritating.

- Always stay calm and do not show irritation.

Paranoia and suspiciousness

These are very common. The person with dementia may become suspicious of the carer or of other people. They may feel that people are talking about them, being malicious behind their back. Or they may think that people are stealing from them. They may suspect that their partner is being unfaithful or deceitful.

A more severe manifestation is the development of a delusion. These, too, are not uncommon in Alzheimer's disease. They are common in dementia with Lewy bodies and can also occur in Parkinson's disease dementia. A delusion is a false belief that cannot be reasoned away – for example, believing that there is someone locked in a cupboard or that their grandfather is still alive.

Paranoia is the misbelief that people are talking about or conspiring against you. It may simply be a suspicion or it can be a paranoid delusion, when they become convinced that this is the case despite a lack of evidence.

TIPS FOR DEALING WITH SUSPICIOUSNESS OR PARANOIA

- Don't react or be offended. The dementia is causing this – it is not a thought-out conclusion.
- Arguing will stoke up the emotion and make the person distressed.
- Offering a logical explanation might help.
- Try to distract the attention onto something else.

Disinhibited behaviour

The person with dementia in this middle stage may start to exhibit bizarre behaviour, which seems antisocial, rude or offensive. They may lose any sense of propriety, which can cause embarrassment to the family and carers. They may be rude to other people, becoming insensitive to other people's feelings. They may be sexually aroused and attempt to kiss, cuddle or fondle other people. They may expose themselves in public.

TIPS FOR DEALING WITH DISINHIBITED BEHAVIOUR

- Try to understand what triggers it. If you can then you may be able to avoid those circumstances.

- There may be a physical reason, so check with the doctor so as to exclude this.
- React calmly and do not react physically. Do not coerce them or tell them off, as that may make matters worse.
- They may be doing this because they have become confused or they may have mistaken someone else for a loved one. Persuade them to go to another place or another room and distract them by doing some activity. If they have been exposing themselves or touching someone else, then gently tell them that it is not appropriate.
- They may feel in need of attention, so try to be calm and reassuring. They may respond to patting or stroking.
- If someone repeatedly exposes themselves then consider getting clothing that they cannot easily remove without help.

Wandering

This is very common. Indeed 60 per cent of people with dementia will wander at some point. This is because they easily get disorientated and forget their address and may think that they are going to go back to somewhere else – an old house they once lived in, for example.

Outside their own environment they get even more disorientated.

TIPS FOR DEALING WITH WANDERING

- Make the home as comfortable as possible, but do not make it a prison.
- Keep up the daily routines.
- Identify when wandering occurs. It is common at dusk, when the person may get disorientated.

- Don't argue if the person is convinced that they have to go somewhere else, or they believe that they live elsewhere. Instead, be reassuring and perhaps tell them that they are staying 'here' tonight.

- Check that there is not a physical reason for them being confused.

- Night wandering can start because the person wakes up wanting to go to the toilet. Avoid too much fluid last thing at night. Also, use electric nightlights in the home, so that if they do get up they cannot injure themselves.

- Consider having locks moved so that they are not in the usual place on the door.

- Consider the decoration of the rooms. Having doors the same colour as the walls may 'camouflage' the doors.

- Avoid going to busy places, like shopping centres, which may confuse the person with dementia. They can find this very disorienting and the disorientation can persist when they return home and induce wandering.

- Always make sure that there is someone with the person with dementia.

- Consider movement detectors, which will signal if someone has wandered in the night.

Sleep problems

About 20 per cent of people with dementia experience increased confusion, anxiety and restlessness at dusk and throughout the evening into the early hours. They may simply not want to sleep.

This can be exhausting for a spouse or live-in carer who needs to get sleep to ensure they maintain their own health. Fortunately, this night-time restlessness does not last forever. It typically occurs in the middle stages of dementia, then disappears in the late stages, whereupon the person will sleep more.

In general, hypnotics (sleeping tablets) are not used, because they can make matters worse.

TIPS FOR DEALING WITH SLEEP DIFFICULTIES

- Maintain a regular routine throughout the day, with regular bedtime and waking-up times.
- Avoid stimulants like coffee and alcohol in the evenings.
- Consider a milk drink before bed.
- Make sleeping something that will be enjoyed, so make the bedroom comfortable, keeping nightlights on, and ensure that the person has a comfortable bed.
- Have some activities in the day so that the person with dementia has a full enough day that their body and mind is ready for sleep.

Sundowning

This is a pattern that can occur at sundown in many people with dementia. The person with dementia may get confused, anxious, agitated, aggressive or restless. They may experience hallucinations, show repetitive behaviour or start to wander.

About two thirds of people with Alzheimer's disease and other dementias may get this in any stage, although it tends to peak in the middle stage. It then tends to lessen as the condition progresses.

It can be triggered by tiredness, becoming disorientated because of the failing light, or because the main activities have been early in the day, making them restless as sundown approaches.

If it occurs, look for a cause. Is the person in discomfort from something? They could be hungry, or they may want to go to the toilet. Always try to exclude a physical reason that may be upsetting them.

The following may help:

- Allow adequate time for rest including little sleeps between activities.

- Avoid making appointments at the end of the day, typically at sundown when disorientation occurs.

- Try to limit shadows by having bright lighting.

- Keep the person active at sundown and in the early evening.

- Avoid stimulants like coffee or alcohol at sundown.

- Try to maintain routines.

- A rocking chair is worth considering, since it is a pleasant motion, both relaxing and stimulating.

Eating and drinking

These are very important during both the middle and late stages of dementia. People with dementia are at risk of becoming malnourished and dehydrated. This can come about for several reasons:

- Memory difficulty – the person may forget whether or not they have had a meal or a drink.

- Apraxia – the person with advanced dementia may forget how to use everyday objects such as cooking utensils.

- Dysphagia – this means difficulty with swallowing. It is a common symptom in middle and late dementia and the person may avoid eating or drinking because of this.

- Decreased appetite because the parts of the brain dealing with appetite have become damaged.

- Loss of smell and taste because the parts of the brain which receive and interpret sensory information may have been damaged by the dementia process.

- Underlying physical disease unrelated to the dementia may affect appetite.

- Ill-fitting dentures – the person's mouth may have changed as gums recede and tissue is lost.

- Poor oral hygiene resulting in a sore mouth.

- Digestive problems.

- Side effects of medication.

- One's culture and religious beliefs not being taken into account when food is prepared. This has to be borne in mind if someone is in a residential home.

There are a series of tests that doctors and nurses use to assess the individual's nutritional state. If you are concerned about the person with dementia's nutritional state or their level of hydration, then ask your doctor to do an assessment.

TIPS TO HELP A PERSON WITH DEMENTIA TO EAT

- Mealtimes should be at regular times as part of the daily routine.
- Use familiar cooking smells to stimulate the appetite.
- Food should be appetising!
- Eating at a table is to be encouraged, with a neat and clear place setting.
- Use appropriate utensils for the person's culture.
- Make it fun.
- Use appropriate utensils according to the person's mental capacity. If the person has forgotten how to use a knife and fork, they may be more comfortable with a spoon.
- If the person needs help, then maintain eye contact and explain that you are helping.
- Do not be forceful. If they spit food out, be patient and do not get cross.
- Be thoughtful about the way you supply each mouthful. Getting the person to put their hand over yours as you raise the mouthful to their mouth can help them to feel some control and maintain dignity.
- Do not put too much on the spoon or fork for each mouthful.

Dressing and grooming

It is likely that the person will need some help with dressing, bathing and grooming during the middle stage of dementia. Dignity is all-important.

Allowing the person to choose and be involved in how they dress, encouraging them to maintain their appearance and take pride in it, is good for maintaining self-esteem. It is better to keep them involved as much as they are able than to take over the process for them. Breaking the process down into simple and understandable stages can be helpful.

Incontinence

This will become a problem for many people in the later middle stage of dementia and for virtually all people in the late stage of dementia. Incontinence means losing control over bowels or bladder. There are many potential causes, so if it suddenly starts or if it gets suddenly worse and more frequent, ask your doctor to assess.

It is a good idea to have the input of a continence adviser. Your doctor can probably arrange this.

Possible causes of incontinence are:

- Urinary infections

- Prostate problems in men

- Constipation (which causes a blockage which in turn causes 'overflow' of loose faecal waste past the blockage). An enema may make a huge difference

- Prolapse in women

- Stroke

- Diabetes mellitus

- Parkinson's disease

- Medication side effects

- Excess tea, coffee or fizzy drinks that have a diuretic effect (make the individual pass more urine).

- Physical inability to reach the toilet or commode in time.

TIPS FOR DEALING WITH INCONTINENCE

- Do not overreact and do not show irritation.
- Be reassuring, since they may feel extremely embarrassed and guilty.
- Help them to the toilet, but respect their privacy.
- Try to incorporate toilet visits into the daily routine.
- Remind the person to go regularly.
- Maintain their self-esteem and use normal language, not childish words for bodily functions, treating them like a child.
- Learn to recognise the signs that indicate the person with dementia is ready to go to the toilet.
- Do not restrict fluids, since it is important that they remain well hydrated.

A word about the strange emotion of disgust

It seems a valid point at which to talk about disgust. There are about half a dozen basic emotions that appear in a person's early development which are pretty universal across every culture: sadness, fear, anger, happiness, surprise and disgust. Each of these has a distinct and recognisable facial expression. Indeed, Charles Darwin described them in one of the books he wrote after his classic *On the Origin of Species*.

These emotions have evolved over millions of years and each has a useful function. Sadness allows us to adapt to loss. Fear helps you avoid physical threat. Anger pumps up your energy, urging you to overcome an obstacle. Happiness reinforces success. Surprise opens you up to learning. Yet of all these basic emotions, disgust is the only one that concerns your health.

Disgust tends to prevent an individual's exposure to germs, disease or contaminants. When disgusted you screw up your face and you may get an impulse to retch, to expel something from the system.

There are three main types of things that disgust protects against. Bodily fluids are top of the list, because we perceive them to be contaminating; then rotting or decaying food and, lastly, bodily violation. We instinctively dislike the thought of needles, knives and things that could hurt us.

The point is that if you feel disgusted at having to deal with body waste, just accept that this is an instinctive emotion but also that it won't last. As soon as the task is done, it will go, so just put on your apron and your gloves and do it. What you must not do is allow the negative side to dominate. Don't allow yourself to get confused and be disgusted with the person with dementia. The emotion should not relate to them, but to the waste product only.

In Chapter 14 we will look at how you can use the Life Cycle to distract and change your focus, which will be better for both the carer and the person with dementia.

Late stage care

This stage of the disease can last a mere handful of weeks or it can go on for a few years. The person will need 24-hour care. Their memory may be negligible and they may no longer recognise friends or family.

They may not understand what is said to them and they may no longer have speech. Nonetheless, they still have feelings and they may still respond to things like music, a caring touch and affectionate care.

They will need help with:

- Eating and drinking – this has to be done with great care, since they may have difficulty swallowing

- Personal hygiene

- Incontinence

- Walking may be difficult and they may need help with this

- Eventually, they may end up bedbound, so will require total care.

The person with late stage dementia is still the same person that you knew before the disease was diagnosed. It is the disease that produces the shrinkage of the brain and the symptoms that have been progressively altering the person's behaviour and cognitive function.

Spirituality may have been an important aspect of the person's life and maintaining this, perhaps through pastoral visits from a member of the clergy or representative of whatever faith the person belongs to, can be of great personal help and comfort to the person, even in late stage dementia.

It is certainly not a time to isolate the person any more than the disease has already done. Keep up the routines, involve the person in conversations, even if it becomes more a monologue than a dialogue, and keep them involved by showing photographs, reading to them and playing music.

Physical touch can be very comforting, so massaging oils into their hands, gentle massages of shoulders and stroking or brushing hair are to be encouraged.

And do try to keep the appetite stimulated with tasty food in a form that they can manage.

Physical well-being

Much of the care at this stage is focused on the person's physical health. It is important to be ever-vigilant about symptoms suggestive of infection.

- Unaccounted crying out can be due to pain, the cause of which needs to be diagnosed by the doctor.

- Infections of chest or urinary tract need to be treated.

- The person needs to be moved from bed to commode, or to wheelchair, or into the bath. The carer needs to be shown how to lift safely.

- The bedbound person needs to have their skin protected by being kept clean and dry.

- Bedsores need to be avoided by using pads and pillows to cushion body areas on the elbows, heels, hips and back.

- It is important to keep the joints moving, so passive movements need to be made. Your nurse or physiotherapist will demonstrate this.

- Nutrition and hydration need to be maintained.

- Incontinence needs to be handled with care and dignity.

Further options

This stage of dementia should have been planned for. This is where the person's own wishes which were made perhaps years before, in the early stages, can be enacted. It may have been the person's wish to stay at home or to go to live in a residential home when they reached the last stage of dementia. They may already have been living in a residential home, but now need to be in a nursing home equipped and appropriately staffed to care for the person. A nursing home has nursing staff whereas a residential home may not.

It may be that the needs of the person in their own home are not able to be met by the carer. This can be a difficult decision, but it is important to take into account the health of both the person with dementia and their carer. Moving the person with dementia into a care home may be the best option and should in no way be regarded as a failure (see Chapter 13, *Care homes*).

End of life

This can take place at home, in hospital, or in a care home or hospice. Dementia shortens the life expectancy and is currently the third commonest cause of death in the UK. Death from stroke or heart attacks are still commoner.

If the person has made an advance decision (see Chapter 10, *So I have dementia*), then their wishes about whether or not to have resuscitation in hospital or whether or not to have antibiotics will have been made clear. The medical staff has to accept those wishes.

There may also have been a wish to leave organs for donation or not. They may wish to leave their brain for scientific research. And there may have been instructions about the funeral and burial or cremation. It is all much easier for the family if these things have already been discussed.

Becoming a carer

When someone is diagnosed with dementia, it does not simply affect the individual who has it, but will tend to affect the whole family and whoever finds themselves in the role of carer. Dementia is different from other conditions, being a progressive condition in which the carer may see the individual's personality change and their mental function diminish until they are no longer recognisable as the person they once were.

Becoming a carer for a person with dementia can be painful, distressing and exhausting. As we shall see in Chapter 14 (*Using the Life Cycle to help cope with dementia*) there are strategies that the carer can use to help. In this chapter we shall focus more on the role of the carer.

Carer's assessment

A carer's assessment can be requested if the person that needs caring for is eligible for social services help. The aim of this is to assess what support the carer needs in order to maintain their own health and well-being. This can include needs regarding education, attendance at courses, or relate to their work and their ability to have time to have a job.

Carers Direct

This official website is a treasure trove of information that can help a carer in the UK get support.

There you can find information about:

- Your rights
- Benefits

- Direct payments

- Leaving work or returning to work or education

- Advice on getting a carer's assessment

- Housing issues

- Home care.

Call the Carers Direct helpline on **0300 123 1053** if you need help with your caring role and want to talk to someone about the options available to you. The helpline is open Monday to Friday 9 a.m.–8 p.m. and Saturday and Sunday 11 a.m.–4 p.m.

Keep a diary

When one begins caring it can seem very confusing. It is important therefore to try to establish a routine based upon the person with dementia's needs. A useful thing to do is to keep a diary over a week so that you can chart the tasks that need doing, when and where they get done, and how much time they take. The aim of this is not to weigh yourself down with tasks, but to see what you can do to help the person you are caring for in maintaining their independence.

It may help you to see the sorts of things that aids could help with, or what sort of assistance would help. For example, the person you are caring for may need walking frames if there is a mobility issue, or white boards if notes need to be left to jog the memory.

Continue to work with the community team

The person with dementia may have physical problems or disabilities. This can certainly be the case if someone has vascular dementia. It may be that the problem started after a stroke, so the additional problems of caring for a stroke victim have to be taken into account and addressed. Once the patient is at home the stroke team will probably keep in touch for a while before handing on care to the community team. It is important that the carer has been shown how to lift effectively and safely, if the stroke survivor needs such help. This you will be shown how to do by the physiotherapist and occupational therapist.

The GP will be the person that you liaise with in the community team. They will look after the individual's medical care and mobilise whatever further assistance is needed. This may include help from:

- A nurse practitioner or practice nurse

- An Admiral Nurse, if there is one in your area

- A district or community nurse

- A continence adviser

- A physiotherapist

- A health visitor

- A pharmacist

- A social worker.

Look after yourself

Very often a carer – whether a husband, wife, sibling or child – will end up taking on many other tasks, such as cooking, bathing, lifting, organising finances and overseeing the administration of medication. This can be physically demanding and emotionally draining. It is important, therefore, to allow yourself free time as well as adequate time to eat and sleep.

Stress can be a problem for carers, so it is useful to seek advice from your GP if you develop a sleep problem, experience anxiety attacks or develop any physical symptoms. A lot of people don't admit to feeling stressed, yet whenever they get the chance of some time to themselves, they feel the benefit. Some people regard it as a sign of weakness to admit to feeling stressed, but that is certainly not the case.

It is also as well to be aware of the coping mechanisms you may be using to ease stress. For example, some carers lean on habits or coping mechanisms that may be injurious to their health. Smoking and drinking are obvious ones, but so too are things like gambling, eating junk food or becoming less active. In other words, some coping mechanisms are better than others. Better coping mechanisms may be getting out for a walk, having time to play golf, listening to music or working in the garden.

Daycare and respite care

Since caring can be physically, emotionally and psychologically draining, daycare may have been organised as part of a package of care. For a stroke survivor this is usually in a residential or nursing home, depending upon how much care the person needs.

Respite care is effectively a longer period of care for a week or two in a residential or nursing home or a local hospital. If it is available then take the opportunity for some free time while the person with dementia is being cared for by others in the residential home or other place. It is a time to rest, catch up on your own interests or do whatever you need to recharge the batteries.

Stroke clubs

Stroke clubs are very helpful for stroke survivors to attend, if they are locally available. They give the carer some regular time off from caring, so that they can get on with other tasks and be relieved from the continuous round of duties that come with caring for someone. They are also of great benefit to the stroke survivor, since they offer a social outlet where rehabilitation can continue. And if the person has started to develop vascular dementia, this can be of even more value to the carer.

Carers' groups

Carers' groups may also be available where a carer can meet other carers, share experiences and feel supported. It is often very useful to talk to other people who are carers and find out how they cope with stress and some of the issues like incontinence or repetitive behaviour. You may find that you pick up a lot of useful tips about being positive and how you can help the person with dementia.

Dementia cafes

As we saw in Chapter 9, these are organised by the voluntary sector, including Alzheimer's Society and Age UK. They provide comfortable and supportive environments, a sort of cafe setting, for people with dementia and their carers to meet and socialise. Qualified staff and trained volunteers provide support and information, arranging talks and other activities.

Chapter 12

Medical treatment

Despite ongoing research into the pathology of dementia, at the current time there is no treatment that can cure it. Having said that, there are drugs that can slow down the progression of Alzheimer's disease.

Since vascular dementia has a different pathology and is caused by circulation problems that produce ischaemia (as outlined in Chapter 5, *Vascular dementia*), these drugs are not currently licensed for use in vascular dementia. Drug treatment of vascular dementia will therefore be limited to treatment of the underlying circulation problem. If, however, the diagnosis is of mixed dementia, when Alzheimer's and vascular dementia are both present, then it is possible that disease-retarding drugs could be prescribed.

Cognitive enhancers

These are the drugs that may be prescribed in Alzheimer's disease to try to improve cognitive function.

Acetylcholinesterase inhibitors, ACEIs

These drugs work by slowing down the action of an enzyme called acetylcholinesterase, whose function is to break down acetylcholine (ACh), one of the neurotransmitters that transmit messages between nerve cells. Acetylcholine is vital in the maintenance of memory and other cognitive functions, but in Alzheimer's disease there is a loss of nerve cells and a diminishing amount of this crucial neurotransmitter. The drugs stop the enzyme, thereby allowing more acetylcholine to continue passing messages between cells.

There are three drugs in this group:

- **donepezil** (Aricept)

- **galantamine** (Reminyl)

- **rivastigmine** (Exelon).

The bold letters show the generic names of the drugs or the drug's actual name. The names in brackets are the brand names.

Rivastigmine is also licensed to treat mild to moderate Parkinson's disease dementia.

The ACEIs may help to reduce the hallucinations experienced by people with Lewy body dementia. They are also generally well tolerated, though possible side effects are:

- Nausea

- Headache

- Stomach pains

- Vomiting

- Loss of appetite

- Diarrhoea

- Increased agitation

- Aggression.

NMDA receptor antagonists

This group of drugs blocks the effects of glutamate. Currently, there is one drug of the group that is licensed for the treatment of mild to moderate Alzheimer's disease.

Glutamate, as we saw in Chapter 2 (*Understand the brain*), is the main excitatory neurotransmitter in the brain. It is involved in memory, thinking and learning. However, it has been also found that too much glutamate overstimulates the cells. This happens because glutamate allows calcium to flow into the nerve cells. This produces 'overexcitation', which has been found to lead to cell degeneration and cell death. This is one of the theories as to the cause of Alzheimer's disease, which we looked at in Chapter 4.

Memantine

This drug works by inhibiting another neurotransmitter called N-methyl-D-aspartate, known as NMDA. It is recommended for helping with memory and cognitive function in moderate Alzheimer's disease if the person cannot tolerate the ACEIs. It can also be used in late stage Alzheimer's disease.

It works by blocking the NMDA receptors in the brain. This effectively blocks the excitatory neurotransmitter glutamate, which causes damage to nerve cells in the brain. So its effect is to limit further damage.

Possible side effects are:

- Dizziness

- Confusion

- Aggression

- Depression

- Headache

- Sleepiness

- Diarrhoea

- Constipation

- Nausea

- Vomiting

- Weight gain

- Back pain or other muscle pains

- Cough

- Shortness of breath

- Hallucinations (seeing things or hearing voices that do not exist).

Cognitive enhancers are prescribed in the first instance by a specialist and then continued by the GP. The patient's heart needs to be checked before they are prescribed, since they are not indicated in people with heart problems, especially slow heart rates.

Once-a-day doses tend to be prescribed, since it is best to keep the treatment simple. They need to be reviewed after three to six months to ensure that the person is deriving benefit from them. Many people experience some improvement if the drug is started early enough. They may seem to recall things better and be better able to manage routine things like preparing food or making a drink.

At the assessment the benefit is gauged at cognitive, global, functional and behavioural levels. About a third of people with Alzheimer's disease benefit from cognitive enhancers and may be prescribed them indefinitely.

The treatment of vascular dementia

The emphasis of treatment in vascular dementia is on preventing further cerebral infarcts that would worsen the dementia. This may mean the use of agents like aspirin. Very importantly, treatment will involve help with rehabilitation after stroke and such measures as can, as far as possible, maintain the well-being and independence of the individual.

Aspirin

Aspirin is antithrombotic. This means that it prevents the formation of thrombus, or blood clot. It is also called an antiplatelet drug, because it stops platelets from sticking together and producing a blood clot.

Aspirin is known to have many beneficial effects. It is a painkiller, an antipyretic (lowers temperature) and an anti-inflammatory drug. More and more research is demonstrating that in low daily doses it reduces the risk of heart attacks, strokes and various types of cancer. Its effectiveness arises because it blocks the action of two cyclooxygenase enzymes, known as COX-1 and COX-2. Both are involved in complex metabolic pathways that produce natural chemicals called prostaglandins.

COX-1 has a protective effect on the stomach. It is also present in the platelets, the very smallest blood cells that clump together and help to produce a clot. This clumping of platelets is generally a beneficial effect in the body, because this is the way that we heal wounds. On the other hand, when it produces a clot inside a blood vessel, it is extremely dangerous.

COX-2 is involved in the production of specific prostaglandins which start the inflammatory process.

NICE recommends that 300 mg of aspirin should be given as soon as possible to patients with an ischaemic stroke, and certainly within the first 24 hours. It should not be given to anyone who is allergic to it, or if they have previously had a haemorrhagic tendency, or if they have experienced dyspepsia while taking it.

It should be continued for two weeks or until discharge from hospital if that is sooner. Then the person should have long term antithrombotic treatment with aspirin or with another antithrombotic drug such as dipyridamole or clopidogrel or ticlopidine.

It may be necessary in some patients with past mild dyspepsia to give a proton-pump inhibitor drug such as omeprazole at the same time.

The dosage of aspirin needed to prevent a second stroke is usually 75 to 150 mg.

Aspirin has lots of potential side effects
It should never be prescribed if the patient:

- Has a history of stomach ulceration.

- Has a history of asthma.

- Has had a haemorrhagic stroke.

- Has any blood disorder or inherited condition which could predispose them to bleeding.

- Has had an allergic reaction to aspirin at any time in their life. In this case there could be the danger of having an **anaphylactic reaction**: a serious, potentially life-threatening allergic reaction characterised by low blood pressure, shock and difficulty breathing. This is a medical emergency.

- Is on drugs such as anticoagulants or other drugs which could interact with aspirin to increase the risk of a bleed.

Anticoagulants

These drugs effectively thin the blood and prevent it from coagulating. They may be used in patients who have had a venous sinus thrombosis, one of the rarer forms of stroke. Generally, their role is in the treatment of underlying conditions which may predispose the individual to clot formation, such as atrial fibrillation.

Warfarin has been the main oral anticoagulant up until recently. It necessitates having a regular blood test called an INR (international normalised ratio) every two weeks to monitor the level of anticoagulation that has been achieved. The daily dosage can then be varied according to the local anticoagulant clinic which does the monitoring.

More recently NICE has approved two other oral anticoagulants, dabigatran and rivaroxaban, in the treatment of patients with atrial fibrillation in order to reduce their risk of stroke. They both work in different ways from warfarin, but they have the advantage of not requiring regular monitoring and dose adjustment. NICE recommends that these two can be used in patients with nonvalvular atrial fibrillation, meaning atrial fibrillation in the absence of a heart valve problem. For patients with atrial fibrillation and a known heart valve problem, warfarin is still the drug of choice.

Cholesterol-lowering drugs

Patients in whom the cholesterol is found to be raised may be offered a statin drug, in addition to advice on how to lower their cholesterol through dietary means.

The statins, or HMG-CoA reductase inhibitors, reduce cholesterol levels by inhibiting the enzyme HMG-CoA reductase which is involved in cholesterol synthesis. They reduce the level of the enzyme in the liver which will result in a decrease in the level of cholesterol. They also increase the synthesis of LDL receptors, which helps them to clear low-density lipoprotein (LDLs) from the blood.

Some people react to statins and develop muscle cramps and an inflammatory condition of the muscles called a myopathy. In its extreme form it can cause a breakdown in muscle tissue, called rhabdomyolysis. Nerve damage is also a rare possibility.

However, most people tolerate statins and even if one statin produces side effects then another in the group may be tolerated well.

Antihypertensives

High blood pressure or hypertension is the commonest cause of stroke. It is a condition that can creep up on one insidiously, so it is sensible for all adults to have regular blood pressure checks. For a lot of people who suffer a stroke it may come as a surprise that their blood pressure has been found to be raised. Lowering the blood pressure to an acceptable level is of paramount importance, so the process will be started in the hospital and continued and monitored in general practice.

There are several different types of antihypertensive drugs and the choice or combination of drugs may depend on age and other medical conditions.

The drug groups include:

- Calcium channel blockers

- ACE inhibitor or angiotensin II receptor blockers

- Thiazide diuretics

- Alpha-blocking drugs

- Beta-blocking drugs.

It may be that a patient needs one, two or three types of antihypertensive drug. If a person has vascular dementia, it is generally the case that one tries to keep the treatment as simple as possible.

Drugs for other mental problems in dementia

People with dementia can experience all the other mental problems that people without dementia can have. Not everything can be laid at the door of the dementia condition.

Depression

Depression can occur in dementia. The person's mood may seem very flat, there may be a noticeably low mood in the early part of the day and there may be a loss of appetite. Depression can also make the cognitive functions worse and thus can seem to worsen the dementia.

If depression is suspected then the GP should be seen, since antidepressants may help. The choice of which antidepressant drug is a matter for your doctor to decide. The dosage might not need to be as high as with younger people, because the individual may be more sensitive to drugs.

Sleep difficulties

These are common. It may be that the person can become very disorientated about time and think that night is day and vice versa. Trying to get into good sleep habits with regular bedtimes is helpful. Things that may provoke insomnia should be avoided, such as alcoholic drinks or coffee at night, catnapping in the day and general lack of exercise.

The use of hypnotics (sleeping tablets) is best avoided, since they may cloud cognitive function.

Hallucinations and delusions

These can occur in Alzheimer's disease, they are common in Lewy body dementia and can also occur in Parkinson's disease dementia.

The ACEIs may help reduce the hallucinations in Lewy body dementia, which can be very distressing for the person with dementia and for their carer. On the other hand, they may not be troublesome to the person with dementia, so they do not necessarily have to be treated.

In Alzheimer's disease and vascular dementia, hallucinations and delusions may be helped by antipsychotic drugs. These are the types of drugs used in schizophrenia. They have to be used with care, however, since many of them have side effects that can cause movement problems similar to the movement symptoms in Parkinson's disease (tremor, shakiness, slowness of movement). Accordingly, they could make those symptoms worse in Parkinson's disease dementia. This group of drugs is best avoided in Lewy body dementia, since there is often neuroleptic sensitivity in these patients (see Chapter 6, *Dementia with Lewy bodies and Parkinson's disease dementia*). A specialist needs to assess and prescribe in that situation.

Agitation and aggression

These are not uncommon and in the past, sedative drugs and antipsychotic medication were given, perhaps too readily, in order to make the person with dementia more manageable. Nowadays behavioural approaches are preferred, and these drugs are only rarely prescribed.

ANTIPSYCHOTICS OR NEUROLEPTICS

This group of drugs is used in severe types of mental distress:

- Severe anxiety
- Severe depression
- Schizophrenia
- Bipolar disorder
- Postpartum psychosis.

They used to be known as the major tranquillisers, although they are not actually tranquillising in their action. They are valuable in conditions where people feel detached from reality, and they work to reduce and prevent hallucinations and delusions. They work by affecting the neurotransmitters in the brain, especially dopamine. There are two types:

OLDER ANTIPSYCHOTICS

These are the first-generation drugs and are sometimes referred to as the 'typical' antipsychotics. They are strong in their action, but have quite marked side effects, including stiffness, trembling and reduction of libido.

Examples are chlorpromazine, haloperidol, trifluoperazine and sulpiride.

NEWER ANTIPSYCHOTICS

These are the second-generation antipsychotics, which have been developed in the last decade. Described as the 'atypical' antipsychotics, they also act on dopamine to block its action, though not to the same extent as the older drugs. Consequently, they have fewer side effects on movement, though the user will have more of a tendency to put on weight and the effect on libido and sexual function may be more profound.

Examples are amisulpride, olanzapine, risperidone and zotepine.

Chapter 13

Care homes

There may come a time when the person with dementia moves into a care home.

In the care home there will be trained staff, often including people with special training in dementia care, who can look after the residents throughout the day and the night. They will be able to offer help with daily living, including help with washing, dressing and providing meals.

The commonest reasons for admission are:

- Because the dementia has reached a stage that makes it too hard for them to live independently.

- Because the person with dementia has other illnesses or disabilities in addition which make it too hard to live independently.

- Because the carer is unwell and/or otherwise unable to look after the person with dementia, even with daily help and respite care. For example, if they have to go back to work or get on with their life in another way.

Types of care home

Residential care homes may be run by voluntary organisations, private individuals, private companies that own several homes or a local authority. There are three types of residential care.

Sheltered housing

Here the resident has their own flat in a block of flats, with access to an onsite warden. These may be suitable for someone in the early stage of dementia if on their own or a later stage if they live with their partner. These can be privately owned or rented from the local authority. It is important to know what the warden is there for, since some are available for the person's needs and others are available only for enquiries about the bricks and mortar of the building with no responsibility for the residents' health.

Residential home

These provide a home setting where the person has their own room and en suite bathroom, with communal sitting rooms and dining hall. Some help may be given with washing, dressing and eating. Some of these homes may have staff with specialist training in dementia.

Nursing home

These provide all the services of a residential home, but also have a qualified nurse on duty 24 hours a day. They should be able to look after any person with dementia who requires full nursing care, for example, if they are bedbound, unable to care at all for themselves and have problems with incontinence.

All care homes are regulated in the UK by the Care Quality Commission, CQC. They will provide a list of care homes in the area and can also provide an inspection report, which will highlight the standard of care given and indicate if there are any concerns (see *Useful addresses*).

When and how the decision is made

This very much depends upon what is best for the person with dementia. The person has to be involved in the discussion, along with the carer, the GP or specialist, and the social worker.

If the person with dementia is able to understand and make decisions, and wishes to see whether a care home would be suitable, they can then request a social assessment. If they are unable to make such decisions, then their guardian or power of attorney, who may very well be the carer, will be involved in the discussion on their behalf (see Chapter 10, *So I have dementia*).

The social services will do the assessment, discussing with the GP and hospital specialist, and pointing out the options available. If a care home is considered appropriate then the social worker may help to find a suitable one. The GP, specialist, district nurse, Admiral Nurse or psychiatric nurse may also have knowledge of local care homes.

The social worker will also be able to determine if financial help is available (see the sections on mental capacity and benefits in Chapter 10, *So I have dementia*).

Choosing a care home suitable for the person with dementia

Not all care homes are suitable for the person with dementia. It is important to make the right choice, since it is the person's future home that is being considered. It therefore needs to be a place where their needs will be met and they will also feel comfortable.

You have to ask a lot of questions when choosing a care home. The following points are worth considering:

Location

Will it be close to friends and family, so that visiting will be easy? Otherwise the person with dementia may become isolated. Similarly, is it near shops so that friends and family can obtain things for the person in the care home when they come to visit?

Is the location in a quiet area or is it close to traffic or a railway line? Is it surrounded by trees and fields? The overall ambience needs to be such that the person will feel comfortable.

Cultural needs

Does the care home suit the person with dementia's cultural background, their religious needs? Will there be people there who speak the same language? Will their diet be catered for?

How are the meal times organised? Is there a choice of food? Can the person eat in their room if they prefer?

Facilities

This is obviously of great importance. The care home has to be a comfortable home for the person, but it should also be stimulating.

It should not just be a place where the person is left to stare at a television all day or to sleep in a corner. Are there entertainments, activities or talks arranged? Can the person join in with arts and crafts? Is there a library? Is there a garden?

The person may still be active and accustomed to going shopping, or they may wish to have an alcoholic drink from time to time, so find out if these things can be accommodated.

On the other hand, while access to activities is important, so too is the person's choice. Can they opt out of some things? Can they watch particular favourite TV shows or listen to the radio when they wish?

At the physical end, is there a lift to access other levels of the building? Are the corridors wide enough for a wheelchair or a Zimmer frame? Are there suitable adaptations for disabled use of the bath or shower?

How dementia-friendly is the building itself? Are there lots of corridors, which may confuse the person with dementia? Are there several toilets? How easily can the person with dementia get to them? Will there be help available to the person throughout day and night if they need help getting to the toilet?

What level of training have staff members had in caring for people with dementia?

Their own room

The person with dementia may like their own space, so can they go to their room whenever they want. Can they bring their own furniture to make it familiar? And can they have guests visit them in their room?

The sitting room

How is it arranged? Are the seats arranged in a circle, which can be intimidating for some people, or are they in small groups, so that people can choose where they want to be and who they want to talk to?

Are there other residents in the care home who have dementia?

What is the cross section of the care home? How well can the care home integrate the person with dementia into the social side of the home?

What is the approach of the care home?

This may be hard to pin down, but is an important question to ask. Basically, is the approach of the home to cater for the individual's needs or is it more rigid, where the resident has to fit in with the organisation of the care home? Ask to see the home's mission statement, which should set out its philosophy and approach.

PERSON-CENTRED CARE

The whole emphasis in dementia care nowadays is on the person and their needs rather than the illness and the problems it causes for the person. Person-centred care has the following principles:

- It values the human dignity of people with dementia and those who care for them.

- It recognises the individuality of people with dementia, understanding that they each have unique personalities and experience of life, which will influence the way the dementia affects them.

- It recognises the fundamental importance of considering and seeking the opinion and perspective of the person with dementia.

- It recognises the importance of maintaining relationships and interactions between the person with dementia and their family and friends, and those involved in their care.

Care plan

A good indication of a patient-centred approach is the individual care plan. This should include information for the staff about ways they can encourage the person with dementia to be involved. It is about giving the staff ways to help the person with dementia to live well.

An important part of this is to treat the person with the respect that they deserve. They should be addressed by the name or title that they feel comfortable with, not given a pet name by the staff, or addressed as 'love', 'dearie' or any other names that the person may find patronising.

They should not be coerced into doing things they do not want to and they should also be allowed to enjoy the facilities of what is now their home. Their personal safety is of paramount importance. So too is ensuring that their health needs are met. They may need help with meals and they may need reminding to drink.

Is there a named member of staff who will be responsible for the resident and who will be most familiar with their current health and their overall experience on a daily basis? A care plan will need regular reviewing.

Medical care

What arrangements are in place if a resident is ill? Which medical practice attends the care home? Are there arrangements for other visiting professionals, such as a podiatrist, community mental health team, district nurse or Admiral Nurse? How are drugs collected and given to the residents? This is of great importance to the person with dementia.

You can always move care homes

Just as one can move home, so too can the individual move care home if their needs do not seem to be met. It is the person's home, after all, so they have to feel comfortable with the place and the staff employed by the care home.

A move is usually done after an assessment has been made. Any change can be very disruptive for a person with dementia, so such a move may need careful planning. The person with dementia should be consulted and their opinion should be listened to. If they are unable to understand, then their relatives need to be involved and once again the need for careful planning of the move is important. It should be done during the day, so that the person does not get unnecessarily disorientated with time. Someone they know should go with them to the new home, so that they can have things explained and be reassured during the move.

If the care home is in a different part of the country, in a different local authority, then there may be issues about funding. This must all be sorted out before any move, since the person's care is the fundamental issue.

Chapter 14

Using the Life Cycle to help cope with dementia

In my own practice I use a model that I call the Life Cycle to encourage patients to examine their life in order to devise strategies that they can use for self-help. I do not pretend that this is any kind of rocket science. It is simply a model that many people find useful in helping them to gain a bit of focus. In fact, it can be useful both to people with early and middle stage dementia and to the carer of the person with dementia.

We will run through it all in this chapter and end by looking at a few examples of how it can be adapted for both the person with dementia and the carer of a person with dementia.

The Life Cycle

This term 'Life Cycle' may take you back to your days of studying biology when you looked at the different life cycles of insects, fish, frogs and other creatures. I am not, however, using the term in the sense of a person's development with age, but in the sense of the different levels or spheres that make up one's life at any given point in time.

There is a cycle involved in the manner in which virtually any chronic medical condition affects a person, whether that is a physical one, a psychological one like depression, or a degenerative one like dementia.

To extend the biology analogy a little further, you will learn a certain amount about fish by dissecting them to look at their internal organs. But you won't know how they move and feed without studying them in water. And you won't learn about their behaviour with other fish and predators unless you observe them in a realistic environment. Even then you will not get to know about them fully unless you become a total observer of them.

So it is in medicine. In order to help someone you need to know as much as possible about their condition, their symptoms and the things that make their symptoms better or worse. And ideally you want to know about their habits, their diet, their desires, their fears, their relationships and so on. That might seem like a tall order, but if you can build up such an all-round picture of the patient, then you can see how a condition is truly affecting them at all levels of their life.

This holistic model enables the individual to build a picture of their whole life as it is affected by the condition, considering five levels or spheres of life:

- Body – physical symptoms, e.g. pain, stiffness, tiredness.

- Emotions – how you feel, e.g. anxious, sad, depressed, angry or jealous of others.

- Mind – the type of thoughts you have, e.g. pessimistic thoughts, negative thoughts, self-defeating thoughts.

- Behaviour – how the condition makes you behave, e.g. isolating yourself by avoiding things or people, developing habits such as smoking or drinking, becoming inactive, hitting out at others.

- Lifestyle – how it affects your ability to do things, your relationships, and also how events in your life impact on you.

Figure 9

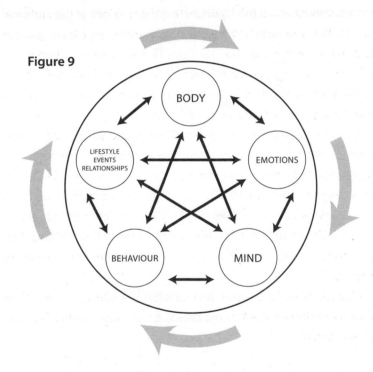

In Figure 9 you will see the five spheres starting with the body sphere at the top and progressing clockwise through emotions, mind, behaviour and lifestyle. The outer circle that encloses the whole structure represents the individual's whole self, their life, and the five spheres all make up the individual's experience of life.

The outer arrows represent the general progression, the Life Cycle, because the order represents the way that a condition will tend to impact on a person and their life. That is, physical symptoms make the individual aware that something is wrong in the body. This can induce an emotional response, which could be anxiety, anger, resentment or fear. The emotions felt alter the way that one thinks and the type of thoughts that you have. This may make you take a particular action or behave in a certain way – to reach for a drink, take a tablet or wrap up – until the emotion goes away. Your actions or behaviours may affect your lifestyle, stopping you doing things, which in turn may affect relationships and work. And all of this can set the cycle off again.

The arrows between the spheres show that every sphere impacts on every single other one; a pain, for example, impacts on all spheres of your life.

On the other hand, importantly, the inner arrows give you the opportunity to use any of the other spheres to reduce the pain or to deal better with it. And you can also see that you are not helpless, that there are all those potential strategies which can help.

Use the Life Cycle to sketch out your life

Get a notebook and make it your Life Cycle diary. Use a double page and draw the diagram on the left-hand page. Draw the five spheres and label them, but leave enough room to jot things down inside them. Draw all of the arrows as in the diagram.

On the right-hand page you can make notes.

In each sphere on the diagram make an entry. It can be fairly simple. Think about how you are feeling that day. The first thing that may come into your mind might be a physical feeling. It may be 'fatigue' or 'backache' or 'sore throat', whatever you are aware of. Write that down inside the body sphere. You can make notes about it on the right-hand page.

With emotions it might be 'depressed' or 'sad'. Jot that in the emotions sphere and on the right-hand page jot down words or notes that describe it better. What are you feeling sad or depressed about?

With thoughts write down the thoughts that you have.

With behaviour write down what actions your emotions and thoughts have made you do. If you were focused on the body sphere of pain, did it make you take a painkiller, or perhaps rub the sore part?

And with lifestyle, did it affect those about you? Did you fall out with anyone? And if you did, did that make you feel happy or guilty or angry or what?

You will soon see that some sort of a pattern manifests itself. You may feel that it would work better if you score every entry, that is, give it a positive or a negative score. That way you can produce a number for each sphere. The emotion sphere and the thought sphere will probably initially have marked negative scores.

You can see that the outer cycle is effectively a chain reaction. Body symptoms create an emotion, the emotion creates a thought pattern, the thoughts make you behave in some way and that behaviour or action impacts on your lifestyle or your relationships, which in turn can affect the body symptoms.

The inner arrows show the way that each sphere impacts on other spheres. By using the other spheres, potentially you can use any one or all of them to reduce the weight of any single sphere. Again, with the example of pain you can see that by focusing on any of the other spheres and doing something different, you will actually modify the pain.

In other words, you can opt to focus on the behaviour sphere, choosing a different behaviour or a different action. It gives you multiple strategies and enables you to break a pattern that keeps you locked into a problem. For example, if you have a chronic pain such as you can get in arthritis, where the body pain makes you feel depressed and the depression makes you think gloomy thoughts. Those gloomy thoughts (such as, I am never going to get rid of this pain) make you reach for a painkiller so that you take too many, or persuade you to smoke (though this will actually make you more likely to have pain, because smoking lowers the threshold for pain). That can affect your quality of life and your relationships, which in turn can make you more aware of the pain. The effect is that you keep repeating the same cycle and thus you get locked into chronic pain.

It is the pattern of repetition that you want to break if you want to free yourself from a continuous symptom that is bothering you. By trying to step away from the pain for a while and concentrating on any of the other spheres, and altering what happens in that sphere, you can see how the inner arrows by their influence on other spheres can result in a change of pattern.

KEY POINTS

- The Life Cycle is a model that allows you to look at the different spheres of life.
- By using it to focus your attention on any sphere, you can alter a negative pattern that may be affecting you.

So, now, let us look at the individual spheres.

The sphere of emotion

The person with dementia can feel the whole range of emotions that they have always been able to feel. Dementia doesn't suddenly stop you from feeling any of them. However, the condition gives rise to specific emotions that come about as a reaction to the increasing difficulty that may be experienced with memory and concentration. For example, the following emotions are common:

- Frustration – about not being able to do things that you used to take for granted.

- Anxiety – this can be fear for the future, fear for your family, fear about losing control of your life.

- Depression – lowness of spirits as a result of the condition.

- Irritability – about having difficulty communicating or understanding. Or it can be irritability directed at others because they seem to be impatient.

- Anger – this can start as a result of being told that you have dementia.

- Guilt – this is common and may come about because you feel a burden on others.

Take anxiety, for example. When you feel anxious there is a tendency to tense up. This tension can be eased using a technique called progressive muscle relaxation, which produces a relaxation response. I will describe it when I come to the body sphere. It is a useful technique that many people with anxiety and depression find helpful. It is also a good example of the way that one sphere can affect another. And if it makes you feel more relaxed, then it automatically affects the other spheres, too.

Moreover, the emotions that are felt are not all negative ones. The person with dementia can still have pleasurable emotions. They can still laugh, feel joy and feel love. These positive emotions make life more enjoyable and so, of course, it is worth aiming at doing things to stimulate this positive side.

The sphere of the mind

This is obviously the most important sphere, yet it is not the only one to focus on. I firmly believe that you need to consider all the spheres and get them working for you. Yet the way that you think is of huge relevance because:

- Thoughts arise from the emotions.

- Emotions arise from thought patterns.

- Thoughts and emotions affect and are affected by the other life spheres.

Thoughts arise from the emotions

The kinds of thoughts you have are determined in part by the emotion you are feeling. If you wake up in the morning and you feel happy, then the train of thoughts that you have is liable to go in a different direction from the train that you will have if you are fearful, guilty, angry or sad.

The emotions do not just turn off by you telling them to change. You have to make them change and one of the most effective ways is by thinking. For example, if you feel angry, you will probably start thinking in a way that justifies your anger. You may start unconsciously finding fault with a relative or partner. Instead of allowing yourself to find fault and thereby justify your anger, you might try to forgive them. Or you can make allowances for them, perhaps by thinking that they had not meant to make you angry.

Try to avoid negative thoughts and negative thinking.

Emotions arise from thought patterns

This is looking at it from the opposite end. Whereas the example I just gave you is to do with thoughts arising from emotions, this time we look at emotions arising from thoughts.

If you have had a tendency throughout your life to feel depressed, it may be because you have a way of thinking that leads to depression. This may be a tendency to view yourself, the world and the future in a negative manner.

- Personal view – you may have a poor image of yourself and feel unworthy, inadequate and not as good as other people.

- World view – you may tend only to see the negative side of things, especially about yourself. You may only see what you have done wrong, not what you did well, and you may take one criticism to heart.

- Future – this may only ever seem bleak and gloomy. It may seem that everything that can go wrong will go wrong, and you may think that it is always because of something that you did.

Now, none of this is at all conscious. It happens automatically and is just the way that some people perceive themselves, the world and the future. But it can be changed; it will just take time.

Thoughts and emotions affect and are affected by the other life spheres

The way that you think and the emotions you feel can affect the things that you do. That is, they can affect your behaviour.

You may, for example, start to withdraw and isolate yourself from people. That can in turn affect your lifestyle, because you are not interacting with other people. You then have more time to dwell on your emotions and the negative thoughts that have caused you to withdraw. Rather than allowing yourself to withdraw, you should try to maintain friends and contacts. Keep going to clubs, have lunch or coffee with friends, and keep as active as you can.

Cultivate optimism

A recent study in Finland, published in the journal *Neurology*,[14] showed that cynics and pessimists are at greater risk of dementia than optimists. Pessimists tend to have a lot of negative automatic thought. Let me give you four examples of such negative thought.

- Filtering – is where the individual filters out all the positives and sees only the negative. For example, despite a good day at work, they focus on the single error.

- Personalisation – whenever something goes wrong, they automatically assume it is their fault.

- Catastrophising – they extrapolate all situations to the worst possible scenario, usually finding a reason for not doing something to prevent a supposed humiliation risk.

- Polarisation – they see everything as two poles, good or bad, black or white, with nothing between.

To think positively, you have to monitor your self-talk and try to alter the negativity. For example, instead of thinking 'I can't do it because I have never done it before,' try thinking, 'It's an opportunity to learn.' Or instead of, 'There is no way this will work for me,' try, 'Let me try to make this work.' Do not accept the false belief that because something happened once it will always happen to you. That actually is not logical. You need to expect it not to happen. Start looking on the bright side and expect good things to occur.

Cultivate mindfulness

Mindfulness is a Buddhist practice which means paying attention to the present moment, deliberately, without judgement. It is a way of experiencing the moment without being sucked into thinking about how it is affecting you or your future, but simply enjoying being where you are. I think it is a useful way to try to induce positive thoughts and positive emotions.

For example, pick any activity of normal life, such as drinking a cup of tea or coffee. Mindfulness would make you focus on the cup of tea, the way that it was made, the taste, the temperature, the feeling it induces. In other words, think of the pleasure that drinking the tea gives you and try to focus on that pleasant feeling. Similarly, with preparing food, think of all the positive pleasures you get as you prepare the food and as you eat it. This is another way of reducing negative thinking, because you are concentrating on the positive thoughts.

The sphere of behaviour

This is all to do with the actions, habits and things that you do. You want to try to avoid the things that cause feelings of poor self-esteem and you want to work against having negative thoughts.

It is very easy for a person with dementia to stop doing things. You can stop reading, stop doing crosswords, stop doing your hobbies or your housework or gardening. Yet staying as active as you can has been shown to be good for someone with dementia.

Doing things requires you to think about what you are doing. And as I mentioned above, if you cultivate mindfulness and think about the enjoyment that you get from doing these things, you will reduce negative thoughts and lift your mood.

The sphere of lifestyle

This is about your relationships with family, friends and acquaintances, the things that you are able to do and the way you interact with people. It is about your home, the things that give you pleasure, your interests, and the things that are part of your life.

You can see how your emotions, thoughts and actions can all have an effect on your lifestyle. Essentially, try to focus on the positives in your life and keep doing as much as you can.

The sphere of body

This is body awareness. Be aware of the positive attributes of the body. Even if you are aware of physical symptoms or if you suffer a physical condition, there are still things about your body that you can enjoy. You need to be comfortable in your own skin. You need to enjoy being you.

Keep active. If you can still enjoy an activity such as walking, or a sport such as playing golf or swimming, then do so. Keeping the body active is known to cause it to release endorphins. These are the body's natural chemicals for reducing inflammation, so they help with painful conditions. They also lift your mood, which is always a good thing in dementia.

Progressive muscle relaxation

This technique is often used in hypnotherapy in order to deepen a state of relaxation. There is no great mystery about it and I recommend it to you as a means of relaxation.

Sit back in an easy chair or lie down somewhere you will not be disturbed by a telephone or other interruptions. Take your shoes off. Close your eyes and just tell yourself that you are going to relax all of your muscles. Tell yourself that as your muscles relax they will become less uncomfortable (use the word 'uncomfortable' rather than 'painful').

Now clench your fists tightly for a count of seven. As you do this, focus your attention on the tightness in the hands, feeling it increase as you count to seven. Then suddenly let it go and tell yourself that instead of tension there is now increasing relaxation in those muscles of the hand. And tell yourself that they will get even more relaxed as you count to 15.

Now clench your fists and this time tense the muscles of your feet, too, by trying to clench the toes. Do this for a count of seven, exactly as before. Then release the tension suddenly and let the relaxation deepen for a count of 15.

Now do it by clenching all of the muscles in your arms and your legs in exactly the same way. Tense for seven and relax for 15.

Then tense all of the muscles in all your limbs, clench the buttocks together, and tense the stomach muscles and your neck and face muscles. Screw your eyes tightly closed as you count to seven, and then suddenly release and relax for 15.

Then tell yourself that your muscles are now going to relax totally, that they will continue to relax and will feel more comfortable when you stop. Now imagine that a wave of relaxation is moving all the way up and over your body from your feet, up your legs, and up your back and chest to your neck. Let that feeling pass down both arms and up your neck to your head, relaxing all of the muscles as it moves up over the top of your head and down over your face.

Tell yourself that you will enjoy this feeling for a minute or so, and if you fall asleep, all well and good. But after the time is up just tell yourself that your muscles feel good; indeed, they continue to feel better and will go on feeling better each time that you do this.

It is as simple as that. And the thing is, the muscles will develop a memory of their own and will get less uncomfortable. Just make it something you do every day.

Putting it all together

I said that this was not rocket science, yet it is a practical model that the person with dementia can certainly use in the early stage of dementia. I think it is a good exercise, for it requires you to focus on the different aspects of life.

It is something that a spouse or carer can do, too. It is done in exactly the same way and provides a means of examining how the person with dementia's condition is affecting you as a carer, giving you a way of looking at strategies you can use to help both them and yourself.

Finally, it gives a carer a plan or a means of working out ways of dealing with behavioural problems or emotional problems that occur. There should always be something that you feel you can do to help.

KEY POINTS

- You don't have to worry about the inner arrows, they just show how one sphere ultimately is linked to every other sphere.
- Just focus on changing one of the spheres and the overall negative pattern may be changed.

Let us look at the example of difficulty getting off to sleep from the point of view of the person with dementia. You would write 'tiredness' in the body sphere. This could make you feel anxious, so the word 'fear' or 'anxiety' goes into the emotion sphere. That starts thoughts about not being able to sleep when you go to bed, so 'Worry about staying awake' goes into the thought sphere. This may make you do certain things, such as take a sleeping tablet or have a drink of alcohol, so 'sleeping tablet' or 'alcohol' goes into the behaviour sphere. This becomes part of your lifestyle as a habit. You have developed the habit of not sleeping. You write 'habit' in the lifestyle sphere. This in turn affects your ability to sleep again.

You see how it can be a cycle that repeats itself. Well, focus on any of those spheres and try to do something different. Try to make yourself feel differently, think different thoughts or do different things, and you may change the pattern. For example:

Emotion sphere – Try to get rid of the fear of not sleeping. This is not as hard as you might think. A fear of this kind is called *anticipatory anxiety*, meaning fear that one has before an event. The anxiety about something happening is actually more likely to make it happen. Thus, if you worry that you won't sleep then you probably will not.

Thoughts – One thing you can do is to use the technique of *paradoxical intention*.

People troubled by insomnia usually go to bed and try too hard to sleep, the result being that they cannot sleep. With paradoxical intention you try to do the exact opposite. That is you go to bed and you try 'not to sleep'. You may be amazed at how hard it then is to stay awake.

What you are doing is thinking in a different way. You are stopping thinking about not sleeping and thinking about how you are going to try to stay awake. Because you are then not thinking about how awful staying awake can be, the fear goes.

Behaviour – You can change the things that you do. For example, make sleep a regular routine, with regular bedtime and waking-up times, regardless of whether you feel tired or not.

Avoid stimulants like coffee and alcohol in the evenings and consider having a warm milk drink before bed.

Lifestyle – Make sleeping something that will be enjoyed and going to bed something to look forward to. Make the bedroom comfortable, keeping nightlights on, and ensure that you have a comfortable bed.

And now from the carer's view

And now let's look at the example of incontinence from the view of the carer.

Incontinence goes into the body sphere. The carer might feel disgusted by the incontinence, since they do not like handling body waste, whether urine or faeces or both. So disgust goes into the emotion sphere. This makes them justify their emotion with resentful thoughts. Into the thought sphere that goes. This makes them brusque in their actions and perhaps demonstrably irritated. This impacts on the lifestyle or the relationship and they become intolerant. The intolerance may affect the person with dementia negatively, so that the incontinence does not improve and a negative cycle is engendered.

But you can see that by focusing on the spheres, you can change what goes into any of them and thereby, potentially, you will alter the pattern. For example, by altering the feeling of disgust that you, the carer, experience (see Chapter 11, *Caring for someone with dementia*) you can modify the way that you behave, and thus you alter the lifestyle sphere, make the relationship better, and thus you are better able to deal with the incontinence.

Chapter 15

What can you do to reduce your risk of dementia?

In Part One we looked at some of the causes of the different types of dementia. For anyone who has a relative with dementia, it is clearly important to know how you can reduce your risk of developing the condition.

Risk factors for dementia

Some of the following risk factors cannot be altered, yet many others can. First of all, let us look at those factors that you cannot control.

Risks you cannot control

Genes

We considered this in Chapter 4 (*Alzheimer's disease*). There are three genes associated with early onset Alzheimer's disease. Altogether these account only for about 10 per cent of early onset cases of Alzheimer's disease and only one in a thousand of all cases of Alzheimer's disease.

If there is a strong family history of Alzheimer's disease, or a history of early onset dementia, then genetic testing may be worth discussing with the GP.

> ### KEY POINT
>
> A strong family history means having a parent, brother, sister or child with dementia.

The specific condition called CADASIL (Cerebral autosomal dominant arteriopathy with subcortical infarcts and leukoencephalopathy) is something of a special case. This rare inherited genetic disorder is associated with frequent migraines and repeated strokes. It starts at a young age, about thirty, and can be diagnosed by blood and tissue sampling. There is no specific treatment, but antiplatelet drugs like aspirin, clopidogrel and dipyridamole may be used to reduce risk of stroke.

Gender
Some types of dementia are commoner in women and others in men.

- Overall, two thirds of people with dementia are female.

- Alzheimer's disease is commoner in females than males.

- Hippocampal-sparing Alzheimer's disease is commoner in males than females (see Chapter 4, *Alzheimer's disease*).

- Vascular dementia is more common in males than females.

- Dementia with Lewy bodies is commoner in males than females.

Race

Vascular dementia is more common in Asian and Black Caribbean people.

Age

The greatest risk factor for dementia is age.

- One in 1,400 people aged 40–64 years have dementia.

- One in 100 people aged 65–69 years have dementia.

- One in 25 people aged 70–79 years have dementia.

- One in 6 people aged 80 years and over have dementia.

- There is a doubling of the risk of getting Alzheimer's disease every five years after the age of 65 years.

Risks you can control

As we discussed in the chapter on vascular dementia, the main risk factor for the development of vascular dementia is stroke. Therefore, all the factors that put people at risk of having a heart attack or a stroke also put them at risk of vascular dementia.

- Hypertension – high blood pressure

- Raised cholesterol

- Irregular heart function, especially atrial fibrillation

- Smoking

- Excess alcohol

- Diabetes mellitus

- Lack of exercise

- Obesity

- Head injury history – either a single or multiple head injury, as can occur in contact sports.

Four important factors that shrink the brain

A recent research study from the University of California at Davis, Sacramento, published in the journal *Neurology* in 2011, concluded that there are four factors in middle age that are liable to cause brain shrinkage and can possibly lead to cognitive impairment a decade later.[15]

These are:

- Smoking

- Being overweight

- Diabetes

- High blood pressure.

The study found that people with these four different factors had greater shrinkage of the brain when compared to people without any of these factors. Interestingly, they also seemed to show slightly different patterns.

- Those with high blood pressure developed white matter change, which indicated small blood vessel damage in the brain.

- Those with diabetes showed greater shrinkage in the area of the hippocampus, associated with memory function.

- Those who smoked had greater overall shrinkage of the brain.

- Those who were clinically obese were more likely to be in the 25 per cent with the greatest cognitive impairment.

- Those with the highest waist-to-hip ratio were most likely to be in the top 25 per cent with the fastest shrinkage of their brains (waist-to-hip ratio gives a measure of plumpness).

Reduce your risk of dementia by being an optimist

There have been several studies that suggest that people who are optimists tend to have fewer health issues than pessimists. One study at the Mayo Clinic in the USA looked at 1,000 people who had taken the Minnesota Multiphasic Personality Inventory (MMPI), a standard psychological test, 30 years previously. This test has an Optimism–Pessimism scale which grades the 'explanatory style' of the individual. This relates to the way people explain to themselves the events in their lives. Essentially, it categorises people into optimists, pessimists or mixed types. When the review part of the study was done after 30 years, it was found that there were marked differences in survival rates.

The study's authors found that individuals who do not have psychiatric problems but score very high on a personality test pessimism scale have a 30 per cent increased risk of developing dementia several decades later. The same is true of individuals who scored very high on the test's depression scale. The risk is even higher – 40 per cent or more – for individuals who score very high on both anxiety and pessimism scales.

On this basis, they suggested that there appeared to be a dose-response pattern, meaning that the higher the scores the higher the risk of dementia.

As we saw earlier, a recent study in Finland showed that cynics are at a greater risk of dementia than optimists. They studied over 1,500 men and women with an average age of 71 years. They were screened for dementia and given questionnaires to assess their level of cynicism. This included being asked questions such as whether they believed that most people would lie to get ahead or that it is safest to trust no one. After eight years they had another dementia assessment and were asked to take the questionnaire again. During the intervening eight years, 46 people had developed dementia. On looking at cynicism levels, they found that the most cynical and distrustful people were three times more likely to develop dementia than the most optimistic. Being a lifelong cynic therefore seems to be a risk factor, so cultivating optimism is worth doing. We considered this in Chapter 14, *Using the Life Cycle to help cope with dementia*.

Keep up your interests

It has been known for some time that keeping the brain active for as long as you can is helpful in reducing the risk of developing dementia. An American study looked at 200 people between the ages of 70 and 90, all of whom had mild cognitive impairment or had been diagnosed with memory loss, and compared them with 1,100 people from the same age group without memory problems. All of them were asked about their daily activities within the past year, as well as when they were aged 50–65. Those who read books, played games like chess and draughts, did jigsaws, used computers, and did crafts such as pottery, knitting or needlework in their later years were 30–50 per cent less likely to develop memory loss than people who didn't do these kinds of mental activities.

The study also found that people who watched television for less than seven hours a day in their later years were half as likely to develop memory loss as those who watched television for more than seven hours a day. Finally, they found that people who took part in social activities and read magazines during middle age were 40 per cent less likely to develop memory loss than those who didn't do such activities.

The message is clear: you should try to keep the mind occupied with interactive mental activities rather than passive TV watching.

Consider delaying retirement

A French study has recently analysed the health and insurance records of almost half a million people of greater than retirement age.[16] On average those examined were 74 years old and had been retired 12 years. They found that there was a 3.2 per cent reduction in dementia risk for each extra year of work after the age of retirement. That is a considerable figure and may mean that working longer has a real benefit to one's health. There are all sorts of reasons why this may be the case, among which are the social engagement, the mental concentration and the problem solving that occupy you every day at work. Staying at work may just have a silver lining.

Adopt good basic health habits

It seems to be simple common sense that if you adopt healthy habits and avoid ones that are known to be detrimental to health, then you are likely to maximise your chances of staying well. We know that this certainly is true with regard to protecting against cancer, heart disease and stroke, but whether it does so against dementia and a reduction of cognitive function was until recently less well known. Then a large study was done in Cardiff, led by Professor Peter Elwood of Cardiff University,[17] which suggests very strongly that good lifestyle choices help. Researchers had followed 2,235 men for 35 years after their recruitment to the trial in 1979. During the period of the trial the incidence of heart disease, diabetes, cancer and death were recorded. And in 2007 so was cognitive function.

They looked at five lifestyle behaviours:

- Not smoking

- Healthy diet

- Low alcohol intake

- Regular exercise

- Healthy body weight.

They showed that when four out of the five factors were consistently adhered to, there was a reduction in risk of developing dementia of 60 per cent. There was also a reduction in risk of developing heart disease and stroke of 70 per cent. And of the five, exercise was found to be the most effective measure in reducing the risk of dementia.

Get into a good sleep pattern

It is well known that people with dementia often do not sleep well. Whether poor sleep can be a risk factor for dementia is another area that is currently under research, but the evidence does seem to be that good sleep seems to lessen one's risk of developing the condition.

Two pieces of research, in particular, are worth mentioning. The first one is a study of 70 older adults with an average age of 76 years, enrolled in the Baltimore Longitudinal Study of Ageing.[18] The study found that those who slept for less than five hours a night or who had poor, fitful sleep all had higher levels of beta amyloid in their brains than those who had seven or more hours of sleep. Deposits of beta amyloid in the brain, as we saw in Chapter 4, are characteristic of Alzheimer's disease.

The second piece is an animal study on mice, carried out by researchers at the University of Rochester Medical School in New York. They found that during sleep the cells in the brains of mice shrank, creating more room for the flow of cerebrospinal fluid through the brain. It seems that this is a self-cleaning process, clearing out brain toxins such as beta amyloid. The implication is that insufficient sleep may lead to a build-up of these toxins, which may be why increased levels of beta amyloid are found in the brains of people who do not sleep well.

There still remains the question of whether insufficient sleep causes build-up of beta amyloid or whether higher levels of beta amyloid cause less sleep. More research is needed, but it does look as if poor sleep can be a risk factor. In any case, it makes sense to try to get into good sleep habits.

Eat fish

The latest research suggests that eating fish is a good way to stop your brain from shrinking. Previous studies on fish consumption from the University of Pittsburgh have shown that eating fish regularly three times a week reduces the risk of Alzheimer's disease. Now, new research published in the journal *Neurology*[19] has looked at blood levels of omega-3 fatty acids, the 'good' fats in fish, and found that people with higher levels had larger brains than those with the lowest levels.

Brain shrinkage is associated with memory deterioration and a reduction in thinking skills. It is a normal pattern of ageing to get some brain shrinkage, but in Alzheimer's disease this becomes very exaggerated. The study looked at 1,111 women with an average age of 70 years, all enrolled on the Women's Health Initiative Memory Study. All of them had omega-3 levels measured in their blood at the start of the study. In particular, they looked at two types of omega-3 oils, eicosapentaenoic acid, EPA, and docosahexanoic acid, DHA.

Eight years after the start of the study they were all given MRI scans of the brain to assess brain volume. It was found that those with higher levels of these two types of omega-3s had larger brain volume than those with low levels. Interestingly, the brain volume was particularly well preserved in the hippocampus area, a part of the brain crucial for memory function.

Earlier research had shown that people who ate fish regularly had not much more than half the risk of developing Alzheimer's disease compared with those who did not eat fish. The research suggests the important elements in fish for preserving brain volume are these two fatty oils, EPA and DHA.

Omega-3s are found in oily fish such as salmon, trout, sardines and mackerel. They are also found in flaxseed oil and some leafy green vegetables. Eating these at least three times a week may well help you preserve your brain and your memory.

Finally, it is not all doom and gloom

Dementia is a difficult condition to deal with, but it is not all doom and gloom. There may be many years of life when the person with dementia can still live happily and well. The early stage can be a time when you can still enjoy a social life, appreciate books or cinema, play golf or go swimming. The middle stage is also a time, which may last for years, when life can be enjoyed with family and friends. And even in the late stage with care and attention you can be comfortable and feel cared for. Everyone is unique, with their own personality and their own qualities. Aim to enjoy life, both as a person with dementia and as a carer.

Being given a diagnosis of dementia is a life-changing event and marks the beginning of a journey. You can think of it as being akin to setting off downriver in a canoe. There is no map in the canoe, yet you know that many people are all travelling down similar rivers towards their destination. The journey, like the river, can move smoothly at times and at others it may seem you hit rapids and have to deal with turbulent times, upsetting times. Yet you are not alone in the canoe. The person with dementia and the carer are on the journey together, sharing the burden.

And that is one of the things that can help in the journey that dementia takes you on – people. Keeping social contact with others and accepting help whenever it is offered can help you to deal with dementia. As such, I hope that this book has given you, whether a person with dementia, a relative or a carer, information to help you understand the condition, and some strategies to help the person with dementia to live well.

Appendix

Bereavement

When someone with dementia dies, some carers feel that much of their grieving has happened during the years they have cared for their loved one. This anticipatory grief, as it is known, is common in carers of people with both dementia and those with a terminal illness. There may be a feeling of having to put on a brave face and not showing your feelings to the person with dementia, but that doesn't mean that you should bottle them up entirely. Having a good support network of friends and professionals that you can talk to, such as your GP or dementia nurse, can be of considerable help.

Moreover, every situation and every person being unique, some carers will go through the entire grieving process only once the person with dementia has died. It is useful to look at this, since the death of the person to whose care years may have been devoted may seem to leave a huge hole in the carer's life.

The following are the normal stages of grief:

Initial shock

The person cannot accept that their loved one has gone; they may even exhibit the mental mechanism of 'denial' whereby they refuse to believe that the person has died. This shock is often accompanied by emotional blunting, so that the carer does not weep as much as they would expect, or they just cannot cry.

Yearning

This comes after a few days. The person yearns and wants the deceased person to come back. They find themselves filled with memories and images. They want to be close to their things and personal effects. In this period, which can last for a week or two, there is often anger that the person has been taken away, that certain people did not do enough, etc. – anger that is usually unjustified. Then there is guilt, as perhaps the person feels that if only they had done certain things the individual would still be with them. There may also be guilt about things that had not been said before the person died.

Despair

This can last a few more weeks. This is the sadness that comes when they realise that the loved one has gone. It is common for people to hibernate, to become apathetic and to feel that life is pointless. But all this will pass.

Recovery

As the main hurting starts to go, the person will begin coming to terms with their loss so that they can start to rebuild their life.

After three months or so the individual can expect to see some return of joy. Watching a TV show may induce a laugh, or a hug from a friend or relative may make them feel better. If not then the grief may have developed into depression. In particular, if the person starts having thoughts about suicide, or if they feel racked with guilt, then they may need help.

Things that may help one to grieve

It is helpful to try to maintain some sense of normality in one's life during grief or loss. People usually offer help initially, but if their help is declined they may not offer it again. One should try not to be reticent but accept help when it is offered and, indeed, not be afraid to ask family and friends.

Try to get into a routine every day. If you fall into a chaotic pattern of life then it is easy to lose purpose, and losing a sense of purpose can result in depression.

Try not to resort to alcohol, as it doesn't help. It is easy to become dependent on it and to develop a habit that ultimately you do not need and which may contribute to any depression.

Accept that the emotions you are feeling are normal, and if you feel like weeping allow yourself to do so. There is nothing wrong with crying.

Look after yourself and make sure that you get some exercise and have regular nutritious meals, both of which will help.

Glossary

acetylcholine – one of the main neurotransmitters in the brain. Levels are reduced in Alzheimer's disease.

alienist – an old name for a psychiatrist or psychotherapist.

Alzheimer's disease – the commonest form of dementia.

ataxia – a type of movement disorder or stagger.

axon – a nerve fibre which emanates from a neurone (nerve cell), and which conducts nerve impulses.

Benson's syndrome – another name for posterior cortical atrophy.

beta amyloid – a waxy, translucent substance composed of protein, deposited in the brain in dementias, producing senile plaques.

Binswanger's disease – one of the rare forms of dementia due to small blood vessel damage to the white matter of the brain. Today we know it as subcortical dementia.

Charles Bonnet syndrome – syndrome in which some people with sight loss (about half of people with macular degeneration) experience visual hallucinations.

confabulation – making things up to fill in gaps in memory.

delusion – a false belief that is fixed and that a person cannot be persuaded out of.

depression – persistent lowness of mood. But note that in dementia the lowness of mood may not be apparent.

diabetes mellitus – a disorder of carbohydrate metabolism from too little insulin or from a lack of response to the body's own insulin.

disinhibition – the loss of control of one's impulses. People with dementia may become disinhibited and do or say things that are socially inappropriate.

diurnal variation – a tendency to feel most depressed at the start of the day, but gradually improving as the day goes on.

electrocardiogram or ECG – a test to measure the electrical activity of the heart.

electroencephalogram or EEG – a test to measure the brain waves.

hallucination – a perception arising without an external stimulus; may be auditory (hearing voices), visual (having visions) or somatic (imagining body sensations).

hemianopsia – a visual disturbance in which half the visual field in each eye is affected. A stroke is usually the cause.

hippocampal-sparing Alzheimer's disease – a variant of Alzheimer's disease in which the hippocampus is spared. Memory loss is not a feature of the condition; instead there tend to be behavioural problems.

hippocampus – part of the midbrain that deals with memory. It is usually affected in Alzheimer's disease.

hypothyroidism – underactive thyroid gland function.

incontinence – losing control over bowels or bladder.

ischaemia – tissues being deprived of oxygen.

ischaemic stroke – a stroke that is caused by a disruption of the blood supply to the brain by a blockage from a thrombus or an embolism.

lacunar infarction – a specific type of death of brain cells, caused by blockage of a small, deep-brain artery. It results in a melting away of brain tissue to produce a hole, like the hole in a sponge.

myelin – the insulating substance that covers the axons of neurones.

myxoedema – another term for hypothyroidism.

neurone – the basic functional cell of the nervous system, transmitting information by an electrochemical process.

nystagmus – a condition where the eyes move from side to side continuously.

paranoia – the misbelief that people are talking about or conspiring against you.

parenteral nutrition – feeding by intravenous means.

posterior cortical atrophy – a variant of Alzheimer's disease, mainly affecting the posterior parts of the brain.

psychosis – a major mental disorder in which the patient becomes detached from reality.

tau – a protein essential for maintaining the shape of the neurone.

Directory of useful addresses

Action on Elder Abuse

Action on Elder Abuse (AEA) works to protect, and prevent the abuse of, vulnerable older adults.

Tel: 0808 808 8141

Website: www.elderabuse.org.uk

Age UK (formerly Age Concern and Help the Aged)

Age UK is one of the UK's leading charities for the elderly. It provides life-enhancing services and vital support to many people with dementia. Age UK also has many dementia group meetings throughout the UK; a group can be found in almost every county.

Tel: 0800 169 6565

Website: www.ageuk.org.uk

Alzheimer's Society

The society is dedicated to supporting people with dementia and their families, and provides:

- Practical and emotional help such as helplines and support groups
- Information
- Training for carers and professionals

- Services such as respite care.

Devon House
58 St Katharine's Way
London E1W 1LB
Helpline: 0300 222 11 22
Reception: 020 7423 3500

Fax: 020 7423 3501
Website: www.alzheimers.org.uk
Email: enquiries@alzheimers.org.uk

Brains for Dementia Research Coordinating Centre
Brains for Dementia Research is an initiative funded jointly by Alzheimer's Society and Alzheimer's Research UK to address the shortage of brain tissue from individuals that have been assessed regularly during life, which is so essential for research into dementia. Their aim is to lay the foundations for enabling the highest-quality dementia research, with the purpose of finding treatments that will manage symptoms, halt disease progression and ultimately cure dementia.

Wolfson Centre for Age Related Diseases
King's College London
St Thomas Street
London SE1 1UL
Tel: 020 7848 8377
Website: www.brainsfordementiaresearch.org.uk
Email: bdr.office@kcl.ac.uk

Care Quality Commission (CQC)
This body regulates, inspects and reviews all adult social care services in the public, private and voluntary sectors in England.

National Correspondence
Citygate
Gallowgate
Newcastle upon Tyne NE1 4PA
Tel: 03000 616161
Website: www.cqc.org.uk
Email: enquiries@cqc.org.uk

Citizens Advice Bureau CAB
Citizens Advice Bureau aims:
• To provide the advice people need for the problems they face.
• To improve the policies and practices that affect people's lives.
• The service provides free, independent and confidential advice. Advice by phone is available from all CABs and a national phone service is in development.

For Wales call 03444 77 20 20
For England call 03444 111 444 or check your local bureau's contact details
Text Relay users should call 03444 111 445
For Scotland call 0808 800 9060

CJD Support Network
The CJD Support Network was established in 1995 by relatives of people who have died of CJD and is now recognised as the leading charity for all forms of the disease. It offers support to individuals and families affected by all forms of CJD.

PO Box 346
Market Drayton
Shropshire TF9 4WN
Helpline: 01630 673 973
Tel: 01630 673 993
Website: www.cjdsupport.net

The Dementia Action Alliance
This is a movement with one simple aim: to bring about a society-wide response to dementia. It encourages and supports communities and organisations across England to take practical actions to enable people to live well with dementia and reduce the risk of costly crisis intervention.

You can search for your local alliance on: www.dementiaaction. org.uk/local_alliances

Or find the regional lead covering your area at: www. dementiaaction.org.uk/contact/regional_leads

Dementia Friends
This is a national initiative by Alzheimer's Society, aiming to improve people's understanding of dementia and its effect. Anyone can become a Dementia Friend. Just log onto the website and get a free pack and, if you wish, register as a Dementia Friend.

Website: www.dementiafriends.org.uk

Dementia UK
Offers free confidential advice and support on any aspect of dementia care. Their Admiral Nursing DIRECT helpline, staffed exclusively by Admiral Nurses, can offer specialist practical and emotional support

if you're dealing with a diagnosis, worried about your memory or the memory of a loved one, or if you are a professional carer for a person with dementia.

2nd Floor, Resource for London
356 Holloway Road
London N7 6PA
Tel: 020 7697 4160
Fax: 0845 519 2560
Website: www.dementiauk.org
Email: info@dementiauk.org

Department for Work and Pensions
The Department for Work and Pensions (DWP) is responsible for welfare, pensions and child maintenance policy. As the UK's biggest public service department it administers the state pension and a range of working-age, disability and ill-health benefits to over 22 million claimants and customers.

DWP is a ministerial department, supported by 13 agencies and public bodies.

Website: www.gov.uk/government/organisations/department-for-work-pensions

Disabled Living Foundation
DLF is a national charity that provides impartial advice, information and training on daily living equipment. It also provides information about equipment to help with memory.

Ground Floor, Landmark House,
Hammersmith Bridge Road,

London W6 9EJ
Helpline: 0300 999 0004
Tel: 020 7289 6111
Website: www.dfl.org.uk
Email: helpline@dlf.org.uk

DVLA

The Drivers and Vehicle Licensing Agency provides information about driving, licensing and medical conditions affecting driving. It is the organisation responsible for maintaining, and provides information on all aspects of, driving licences.

DVLA
Swansea
SA99 1TU

Driver Licensing Enquiries
Tel: 0300 790 6801
Textphone: 0300 123 1278
Fax: 0300 123 0784
Fax from outside the UK: +44 (0)1792 786 369
Monday to Friday, 8 a.m. to 7 p.m.
Saturday, 8 a.m. to 2 p.m.

Drivers' Medical Enquiries
Tel: 0300 790 6806 (car or motorcycle)
Tel: 0300 790 6807 (bus, coach or lorry)
Fax: 0845 850 0095
Monday to Friday, 8 a.m. to 5.30 p.m.
Saturday, 8 a.m. to 1 p.m.

The Fronto-temporal Dementia Support Group

Formerly Pick's Disease Support Group, this group is particularly directed towards carers who are coping with behavioural changes in a partner, family member or friend as a result of fronto-temporal dementia.

Website: www.ftdsg.org

Huntington's Disease Association Head Office

The Huntington's Disease Association exists to support people affected by the disease and to provide information and advice to professionals whose task it is to support Huntington's disease families.

Suite 24
Liverpool Science Park
Innovation Centre 1
131 Mount Pleasant
Liverpool L3 5TF
Tel: 0151 331 5444
Fax: 0151 331 5441
Website: www.hda.org.uk
Email: info@hda.org.uk

Lewy Body Society

The Lewy Body Society, established in 2006 in the UK, is the only charity in Europe exclusively concerned with dementia with Lewy bodies. The charity's mission is to raise awareness of DLB for the general public, to educate those in the medical profession and decision-making positions about all aspects of the disease, and to support research into the disease. They have produced a series of podcasts and a DVD about DLB.

Hudson House
8 Albany Street
Edinburgh EH1 3QB
Tel: 0131 473 2385
Website: www.lewybody.org
Email: info@lewybody.org

Macular Society

Macular Society has been supporting people with macular conditions for over 25 years. It provides information in the form of leaflets as well as support via its helpline. In addition, it funds research into the condition.

Macular Society
PO Box 1870
Andover SP10 9AD
Helpline: 0300 3030 111 (Monday to Friday, 9 a.m. to 5 p.m.)
Website: www.macularsociety.org
Email: info@macularsociety.org

The National Council for Palliative Care (NCPC)

This is the umbrella charity for all those involved in palliative, end-of-life and hospice care in England, Wales and Northern Ireland. They believe that everyone approaching the end of life has the right to the highest-quality care and support, wherever they live and whatever their condition. They work with government, health and social care staff, and people with personal experience to improve end-of-life care for all.

The National Council for Palliative Care
The Fitzpatrick Building

188–194 York Way
London N7 9AS
Tel: 020 7697 1520
Fax: 020 7697 1530
Website: www.ncpc.org.uk

NHS Blood and Transplant
Organ Donation and Transplantation Directorate
For information about joining the register to donate organs or tissues you can make contact by post or telephone or by filling in an online form at the website.

Fox Den Road
Stoke Gifford
Bristol BS34 8RR
Tel: 0117 975 7575
Fax: 0117 975 7577
Website: www.organdonation.nhs.uk/how_to_become_a_donor

NICE
National Institute for Health and Clinical Excellence was set up in 1999 to reduce variation in availability and quality of NHS treatment and care. NICE issues evidence-based guidance on the management of various conditions as well as public health guidance recommending the best ways to encourage healthy living, promote well-being and prevent disease. It is funded by the Department of Health.

Website: www.nice.org.uk

Parkinson's UK
This organisation provides information on all aspects of Parkinson's disease.

215 Vauxhall Bridge Road
London SW1V 1EJ
Free helpline: 0808 800 0303
Tel: 020 7931 8080
Fax: 020 7233 9908
Website: www.parkinsons.org.uk
Email: hello@parkinsons.org.uk

Stroke Association
UK charity dealing with stroke in people of all ages. They offer a one-off welfare grant for which a professional (e.g. a GP, social worker or physiotherapist) must make an application. Stroke Association's Stroke Information Service provides timely, accurate and personalised information.

Stroke Association House
240 City Road
London EC1V 2PR
Helpline: 0845 30 33 100 (local call rate) or 0303 30 33 100
Tel: 020 7566 0300
Fax: 020 7490 2686
Website: www.stroke.org.uk

References

1 Living Well with Dementia: A National Dementia Strategy – Accessible Summary, Department of Health, 2009.

2 International statistical classification of diseases and related health problems, 10th Revision, Geneva, World Health Organisation, 1992.

3 York, G.K., Steinberg, D.A., Neurology in Ancient Egypt, *Handbook of Clinical Neurology, Volume 952009*; 29–36.

4 Boller, F., Forbes, M.M., History of Dementia and Dementia in History: An Overview, *Journal of the Neurological Sciences, Volume 158, 1998*; 125–133.

5 2011 Census: Population Estimates for the United Kingdom. Office for National Statistics, March 27, 2011.

6 Souter, K., *An Aspirin a Day*, 2011, Michael O'Mara, 117–125.

7 Fox M., Knapp L.A., Andrews P.W., Fincher, C.L., Hygiene and the world distribution of Alzheimer's Disease, *Evolution, Medicine, and Public Health*, 2013; 1: 173–186.

8 McKhann, G.M., Knopman, D.S., Chertkow, H., Hyman, B.T., Jack, C.R. Jr, Kawas, C.H., Klunk, W.E., Koroshetz, W.J., Manly, J.J., Mayeux, R., Mohs, R.C., Morris, J.C., Rossor, M.N., Scheltens, P., Carrillo, M.C., Thies,

B., Weintraub, S., Phelps, C.H., The diagnosis of dementia due to Alzheimer's disease: recommendations from the National Institute on Aging–Alzheimer's Association workgroups on diagnostic guidelines for Alzheimer's disease', *Alzheimer's & Dementia*; 2011 7(3): 263–9.

9 Benson, D.F. (MD), Davis, R.J. (DO), Snyder, B.D. (MD), Posterior Cortical Atrophy, *Archives of Neurology*, July 1998; 45 (7): 789–793.

10 Meagher, D.J., Delirium: optimising management, *BMJ*, 2001; January 20, 322(7279): 144–9.

11 Solomons, L., Solomons, J., Gosney, M., Dementia and Cancer – a review of the literature and current practice, *Aging Health*, 2013; 9(3) 307–319

12 Brooke, P., Bullock, R., Validation of The 6 Item Cognitive Impairment Test, *International Journal of Geriatric Psychiatry*, 1999; 14, 936–940.

13 Whear, R., et al., What Is the Impact of Using Outdoor Spaces Such as Gardens on the Physical and Mental Well-Being of Those With Dementia? A Systematic Review of Quantitative and Qualitative Evidence, *Journal of the American Medical Directors Association* online, July 14, 2014.

14 Neuvonen, E., Rusanen, M., Solomon, A., Ngandu, T., Laatikainen, T., Soininen, H., Miia Kivipelto, M., Tolppanen, A., Late-life cynical distrust, risk of incident dementia, and mortality in a population-based cohort, *Neurology* online, May 28, 2014.

15 American Academy of Neurology, High blood pressure, diabetes, smoking and obesity in middle age may shrink brain, damage thinking, *ScienceDaily* online, August 2, 2011.

16 Dufouil, C., et al., Older Age at retirement is associated with decreased risk of dementia. Analysis of a healthcare insurance database of self-employed workers, Inserm, France, 2010.

17 Elwood, P., et al., Healthy Lifestyles Reduce the Incidence of Chronic Diseases and Dementia: Evidence from the Caerphilly Cohort Study, PLOS ONE online, December 9, 2013.

18 Spira A., Gamaldo, A., An, Y., et al., Self-Reported Sleep and Beta-Amyloid Deposition in Community-Dwelling Older Adults, *JAMA Neurology*, October 21, 2013.

19 James, V., Pottala, J.V., Yaffe, K., Robinson, J.G., Espeland, M.A., Wallace, R., Harris, W.S. (PhD), Higher RBC EPA + DHA corresponds with larger total brain and hippocampal volumes: WHIMS-MRI Study, *Neurology*, January 22, 2014.